Practice Papers for the MRCGP Written Exam, Paper 1

2nd Edition

Dedications

To Alex, Maddie, Alice, Toby, Fern and Scott

Practice Papers for the MRCGP Written Exam, Paper 1

2nd Edition

Rob Daniels MA MRCGP
General Practitioner
Townsend House Medical Centre
Seaton
Devon

Grant Neumegen MBChB MRCGP DPD
General Practitioner (Non-Principal)
Exeter Primary Care Trust
Devon

Joanna Neumegen BM BS BMedSci MRCGP
General Practitioner (Retainer)
St Thomas Medical Group
Cowick Street
Exeter
Devon

Peter Acheson MBChB MRCGP DRCOG DPD PGCertMedEd
General Practitioner
Claremont Medical Practice
Exmouth Health Centre
Claremont Grove
Exmouth

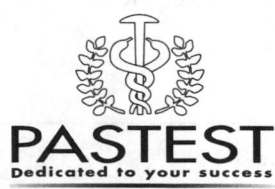

PASTEST
Dedicated to your success

© 2005 PasTest Ltd
Egerton Court
Parkgate Estate
Knutsford
Cheshire WA16 8DX

Telephone: 01565 752000

First edition 2002
Second edition 2005

ISBN: 1 904627 58 7

A catalogue record for this book is available from the British Library. The information contained within this book was obtained by the authors from reliable sources. However, while every effort has been made to ensure its accuracy, no responsibility for loss, damage or injury occasioned to any person acting or refraining from action as a result of information contained herein can be accepted by the publisher or the authors.

Every effort has been made to contact holders of copyright to obtain permission to reproduce copyright material. However, if any have been inadvertently overooked, the publisher will be pleased to make the necessary arrangements at the first opportunity.

PasTest Revision Books and Intensive Courses
PasTest has been established in the field of postgraduate medical education since 1972, providing revision books and intensive study courses for doctors preparing for their professional examinations. Books and courses are available for the following specialties:

MRCGP, MRCP Part 1 and Part 2, MRCPCH Part 1 and Part 2, MRCOG, DRCOG, MRCS, MRCPsych, DCH, FRCA and PLAB.

For further details contact:

PasTest Ltd, Freepost, Knutsford, Cheshire, WA16 7BR
Tel: 01565 752000   Fax: 01565 650264
Email: enquiries@pastest.co.uk
Web site: www.pastest.co.uk

Typeset by Vision Typesetting Ltd, Manchester
Printed and bound in Europe by the Alden Press, Oxford

Contents

Permissions

PasTest would like to thank the following for allowing material to be used in this book:

New England Journal of Medicine

British Medical Journal

British Journal of General Practice

Elsevier Science (*The Lancet*)

Part 1:
Preparation

Introduction

When we decided to write this book we had two goals in mind: firstly, to try to put together a book of practice exam papers, and secondly, to attempt to make it useful as a revision aid. After studying for the exam we felt that none of the books available at that time represented the full scope of the exam, and we all found one of the most stressful aspects was trying to get through all the questions in the time allowed. We felt that a book of questions as close to the exam format as possible would allow candidates to practise against the clock and get an idea of how they will cope.

None of the authors is in any way connected with setting the MRCGP exam. We developed these questions by considering everyday problems we have encountered in general practice and creating questions in the MRCGP style from these situations. The hot topics were prompted by our general reading. Our objective was not to give you an insider's view on what will be in the next exam paper, but to show you the type of questions that might be asked and how to approach answering them in a simple format.

As you look through our questions and answers you will notice that there are simple themes which recur in many questions. There is no secret about passing this exam, all you need to do is have a simple framework around which to build your answers. We hope that by looking through our suggestions you will acquire this skill and soon be able to apply it to almost any question you are confronted with.

When you look at our answers, you will probably think that it would be physically impossible for anyone to write that much in 10–20 minutes. That is probably true, but in developing our answers we have tried to expand the points as comprehensively as possible giving enough detail to clearly illustrate the concepts. We hope that this approach will provide a topic revision aid as well as an answer format – the key really is to look at the headings used for each question and use them as a rough template for developing your own answer plans.

Our answers are not perfect, and we are sure you will be able to think of points we have missed. Everyone has their own slant they like to put on an answer, and with practice you will soon develop your own style. The hot topics questions are derived from current issues we consider to be important and may appear in future papers. There are always more references to find, and you will undoubtedly find those we have missed. The reference lists are for information only. You will not be expected to know page numbers – the publication and year will suffice.

Finally, don't get too worked up over the exam. It is probably the fairest exam you will take in your medical career and if we managed to get merits in the written paper, so can you. Just stay calm, think things through and you'll find you can tackle any topic thrown at you.

Approach to Hot Topics

The thought of tackling the hot topic section of the exam can be extremely daunting, with a seemingly bottomless pit of areas to cover – try not to panic. You are not expected to have an in-depth knowledge of minute detail, more an appreciation of important current areas affecting everyday general practice. What is a hot topic? This is difficult to answer but pointers can be gleaned by flicking through the *British Medical Journal* and the *British Journal of General Practice* and being aware of topical issues arising from your day-to-day general practice. There frequently seems to be a question based on a recent *British Journal of General Practice* editorial, and keeping up to date with topics covered in the 'GP newspapers' can highlight areas to cover. Remember the Paper 1 questions are set months in advance, so don't just consider those topics that are 'hot' close to the exam. Other sources of information include the internet: there are a few good sites, but beware of out-of-date content. Of course an easier way to decide what is 'hot' is to buy a book on the subject, eg the Pastest Hot Topics book. Many of the exam preparation courses include a session on hot topics, although these can be quite expensive.

If you really enjoy studying hot topics, try summarising each key paper into one paragraph. Studying for this section in groups rather than individually can lighten the load and provide moral support. Chatting about topics is often a better aid to memory than reading, and knowledge can be pooled.

When approaching revision for these questions, don't try to memorise too many details. The journal and year are more than sufficient. It is much more important to know the crux of the paper's findings rather than the exact reference. An answer plan is not necessary for these questions, but some sort of structure will appeal to the examiners and help you to process your thoughts. Don't be frightened to write down unreferenced points if you can't recall the source; you may still gain points and it isn't negatively marked.

Critical Reading

The best way to prepare for these questions is to practise in small groups. If you are attending a VTS try staying behind for an hour afterwards in the few weeks coming up to the exam. Each week look at a key paper from the hot topics and criticise it as a group. *How to read a paper* by Trish Greenhalgh (BMJ Books, 2000) is probably the best guide to the subject area. Try to come up with a short checklist of points to consider and use this as a reference when analysing a paper.

Don't be fooled into thinking a paper is perfect just because it is in a peer-reviewed journal. With a little practice, you'll soon spot the errors.

Answer Plans

The key to passing this paper is not knowing everything about general practice, but rather being able to structure an answer plan thinking broadly of areas to cover. This is much more useful than trying to fathom the examiners' construct. When faced with a question about which you know nothing, don't panic. Write down a list of headings and then go through them systematically with explanatory notes. Once you have done a few you will have the bare bones of a decent answer written down and you are nearly there, eg Mr Smith has come for the results of his blood tests showing he has onchocerciasis. What issues does this raise? Starting with simple headings you might get:

Consultation Issues

- Issues for Mr Smith
- Issues for his family
- Issues for the doctor
- Issues for the practice
- Issues for secondary care

Once you have this list, you can start to add to it:

Consultation Issues

- Explore his ideas, concerns and expectations.
- Be honest about own knowledge and limitations.
- Allow plenty of time for questions.

Issues for Mr Smith

- Effects of treatment – may need time off work, may lose income if no sick pay.

- May want to know more about condition, may search internet and challenge GP with this information.
- May want a second opinion.

And so on. As you can see, quite quickly you can build up a reasonable answer. Over time, you will develop your own generic answer blueprint. Some people write it down on a piece of paper as soon as they go in to the exam and use it to plan every answer. Some things are quite useful to try to put in every question, eg Explore the patient's ideas, concerns and expectations; Give advice about support agencies, etc. Others depend on your own personal style. Don't just write these points, though, as the examiners will want to see that you are not just regurgitating headings but that you can put them into the context of the question you are asked. For example, Explore ideas and concerns – Why has the patient presented to you now? Has he read about this illness in a magazine? Is he worried he will become disabled or lose his job? Does he think he has cancer? Is he considering starting a family and concerned about genetic implications? etc.

Topics to Consider Covering

Here's a general overview of some of the areas to consider covering in a plan – definitely not exhaustive, but hopefully giving some pointers on which you can elaborate.

Approach to consultation

- Rapport, empathy
- Ideas, concerns, expectations
- Communication skills – cultural/religious consideration
- Hidden agendas, assess health belief model
- Social/occupational/psychosexual/family context
- Ethics: Consent/confidentiality
- Autonomy, justice, non-maleficence, beneficence
- History
- Examination
- Investigation: Practice-based/specialist
- Management: Check understanding, shared decision making
- Safety netting: Follow-up, leaflets, good record keeping
- Housekeeping: Time management, doctor's feelings/support, eg Young Principals group
- Educational needs – audit, PLP, mentors

Practice/wider issues

- Members of primary healthcare team
- Financial/staff implications
- Care of colleagues
- Professional responsibilities/safety of patients
- Local primary care organisation, eg PCT
- National issues: GP profession – revalidation, morale, recruitment
- Government – funding, rationing, service provision

Part 2:
Practice Papers

Each practice paper contains 12 questions.
Time allowed is $3\frac{1}{2}$ hours per practice paper.

Paper 1

Question 1

The new GMS contract has promised a revolution in out-of-hours care. Discuss the implications of this change for all the stakeholders.

. . . .

. . . .

. . . .

. . . .

. . . .

. . . .

. . . .

. . . .

. . . .

. . . .

. . . .

. . . .

. . . .

. . . .

. . . .

. . . .

. . . .

. . . .

. . . .

Question 2

Mrs Patel, a 40-year-old lady you have not seen recently, attends with one of her children for a routine child health check. You notice she has several bruises at different stages. When you enquire about these, she is evasive. How would you proceed?

. . . .

. . . .

. . . .

. . . .

. . . .

. . . .

. . . .

. . . .

. . . .

. . . .

. . . .

. . . .

. . . .

. . . .

. . . .

. . . .

. . . .

. . . .

. . . .

. . . .

Question 3

As a result of recent MRSA infections in your local community hospital, you are invited to sit on a committee looking into prevention of infection. You wish to make any protocol evidence based.

1   How would you ensure a comprehensive inclusion of data?

Read the extract in reference material 1.1a describing the method of one paper that your research highlights: 'Isolation measures in the hospital management of methicillin resistant *Staphylococcus aureus* (MRSA): systematic review of the literature' (with copyright permission from *British Medical Journal* 2004; 329: 533–539).

2   Comment on the strengths and weaknesses of the database search in reference material 1.1b

3   Discuss the data extraction methodology described in the Method

Reference material 1.1a

Method

Search strategy

We developed a search strategy that covers the main subject areas of the review (MRSA, screening, and isolation of patients and control of infection). We searched the following databases, with no language restrictions: Medline 1966–December 2000, Embase 1980–December 2000, CINAHL 1982–May 2000, System for Information on Grey Literature in Europe (SIGLE) 1980–May 2000, and the *Cochrane Library* to December 2000. We also searched reference lists of retrieved articles and hand searched abstracts from key journals to verify the sensitivity of the search strategy.

Study selection

Two or three reviewers working together appraised abstracts. Full articles were obtained if abstracts mentioned endemic or epidemic MRSA and an attempt at control in a hospital setting.

As the number of studies was far greater than anticipated, we revised the original protocol (which had imposed no quality restrictions). We imposed the minimal requirement that accepted studies should include a component of prospective data collection. If they were entirely retrospective comparisons should have been planned and not prompted by part of the outcome data. No such restrictions were imposed for studies using the most intensive forms of isolation (isolation wards and nurse cohorting) as these have the greatest implications for the allocation of resources and organisation of services.

Two investigators reviewed the papers independently, to confirm that they met the above criteria. We rejected studies not mentioning an isolation policy or without relevant MRSA related outcomes.

Data extraction

We divided each study into phases, where appropriate, that were defined by major changes in isolation or other aspects of infection control policy and extracted data on study design, patient population, isolation details, screening, other infection control measures, and MRSA related outcomes for patients.

We documented potential threats to the internal validity of accepted studies. We considered the vulnerability of each study to selection, performance, detection, and attrition bias (see table 2). We documented measures taken to prevent bias and noted potential confounders and attempts to record and adjust for these. We documented threats to validity because of underlying trends, seasonal effects, and regression to the mean effects, which we defined as 'a tendency for extreme measurements to be followed by less extreme measurements for imperfectly correlated variables that often results in wrong conclusions about the effects of interventions.'[15] We assessed the appropriateness of any statistical analysis undertaken.

We wrote to authors when isolation or screening policies or their timing were unclear. We excluded studies if either the main isolation policy or the timing of interventions were unclear, or if the only outcome reported was MRSA colonisation but the screening policy was unclear or had changed sufficiently to make interpreting outcomes impossible.

Disagreements between reviewers were resolved by discussion and recourse to third parties. Reviewers were not permitted to play any part in appraising a study in which they had participated.

Data synthesis

Two reviewers independently evaluated the strength of evidence in each study by examining the study design, quality of data, and presence of plausible alternative explanations of outcomes. They characterised the evidence on a case by case basis as 'none,' 'weak,' 'of intermediate strength,' or 'stronger.' We considered formal meta-analysis inappropriate because of heterogeneity in outcome measures and patient populations. Full details of the search strategy, study selection, and data extraction are available in a technical report.[16]

Reference material 1.1b

Table 3 Studies providing stronger evidence

Study	Setting and study population	Design	Main interventions	Patient outcomes	Assessment of evidence
Coello et al, 1994[25]	Teaching hospital 1500 beds	Prospective interrupted time series. Three phases: 8, 8, and 26 months	Phases 1 and 2: minimal isolation and screening Phase 3: single room isolation and nurse cohorting, contact screening, prompt discharge of MRSA cases. Topical eradication of MRSA carriage with neomycin nasal cream in phase 1 and with mupirocin in phases 2 and 3	Figure: A 476 infected patients throughout	Evidence that a major outbreak was controlled by combined interventions. Lacks information on many potential confounders
Cosseron-Zerbib et al, 1998[26]	Paediatric ICU 20 beds	Hybrid retrospective and prospective interrupted time series. Two phases: 21 and 24 months	Phase 1: screening for last 11 months Phase 2: single room isolation, cohorting, screening, feedback, handwashing education, barrier nursing, chlorhexidine soap, and other measures	Figure: B MRSA infections: Phase 1: 50 Phase 2: 6	Evidence that interventions reduced MRSA infections. Regression to mean and Hawthorne effects supply less plausible alternative explanations

Table 3 (continued)

Study	Setting and study population	Design	Main interventions	Patient outcomes	Assessment of evidence
Cosseron-Zerbib et al, 1998[26]	Paediatric ICU 20 beds	Hybrid retrospective and prospective interrupted time series. Two phases: 21 and 24 months.	Phase 1: screening for last 11 months Phase 2: single room isolation, cohorting, screening, feedback, handwashing education, barrier nursing, chlorhexidine soap, and other measures	Figure: B MRSA infections: Phase 1: 50 Phase 2: 6	Evidence that interventions reduced MRSA infections. Regression to mean and Hawthorne effects supply less plausible alternative explanations
Duckworth et al 1988,[28]	Teaching hospital 645 beds	Retrospective interrupted time series. Six phases: 4, 3, 13.5, 4, 1.5, 26 months	Initial isolation: mainly single rooms and some cohorting (phases 1–3), changing to mainly isolation ward (phases 4–6). Simultaneous changes to screening, eradication and other measures	Figure: C 408 MRSA infections throughout	Evidence supporting efficacy of combined measures in reducing incidence. Many potential confounders not recorded
Faoagali et al, 1992[31]	Teaching hospital 1200 beds	Retrospective interrupted time series. Two phases: 7 and 8 years Phase 2: overflow isolated in single rooms Additional measures in phase 2 include: pre-screening of admissions and transfers in; handwashing education; antibiotic restriction	Isolation ward throughout Phase 1: minimal overflow from isolation ward	Figure: D	Evidence that combined measures in both phases failed to prevent MRSA spreading and becoming endemic

Study	Setting	Design	Interventions	Figure	Conclusions
Farrington et al, 1998[32]	Teaching hospital 1000 beds	Retrospective interrupted time series. Two phases: 9.5 and 2.5 years	Continual operation of isolation ward Phase 1: minimal overflow from isolation ward Phase 2: overflow cohorted and isolated in single rooms. Screening, ward closure and eradication policies relaxed slightly in phase 2	Figure: E 221 MRSA acquisitions, 206 colonised on admission, 61 uncertain	Evidence supporting control of MRSA for 9.5 years by combined measures followed by eventual control failure related to rise in numbers colonised on admission or to change in strain rather than changed control measures
Harbath et al, 2000,[35] Pittet et al, 2000[36]	Teaching hospital 1300–1600 beds	Hybrid retrospective and prospective interrupted time series. Three phases: 4, 2, and 3 years	Phase 1: No control measures Phase 2: Single room isolation, screening, mupirocin Phase 3: as phase 2 + hand hygiene, education, and feedback programme	Figure: F 1771 MRSA colonisations and infections. 158 bacteraemias	Evidence supporting control by combined interventions. Some potential confounders, but these provide less plausible explanations for the changes

Reference material 1.1c

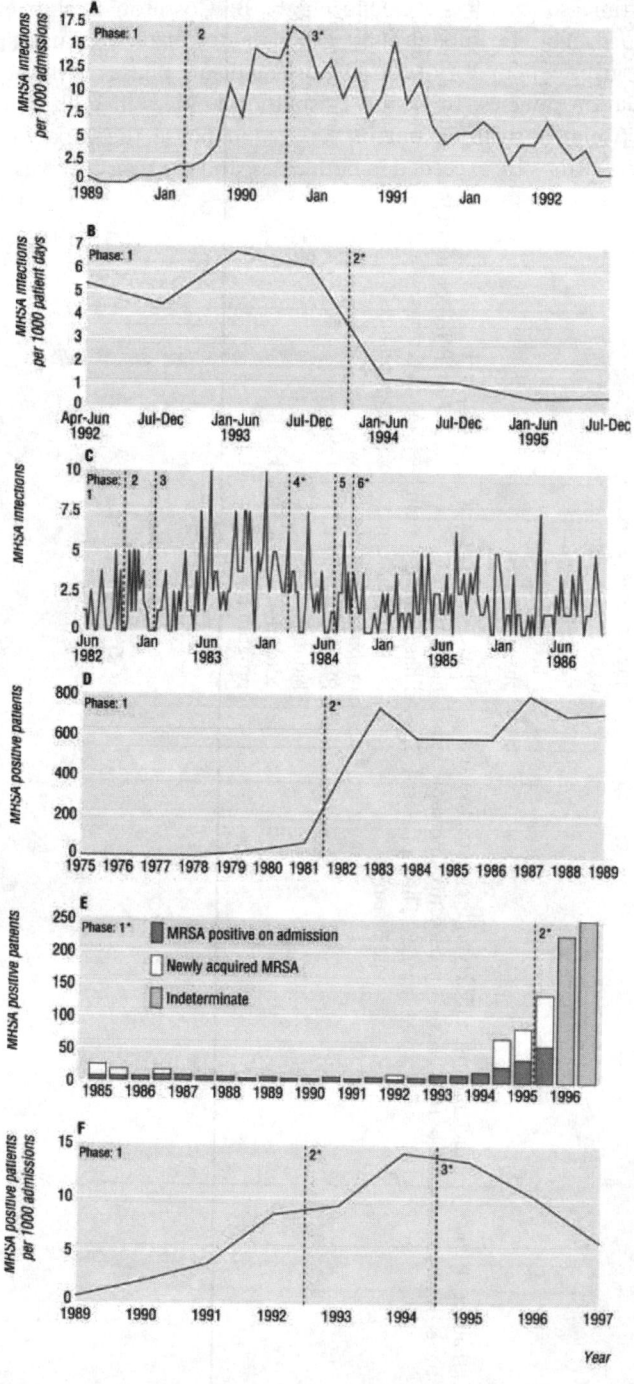

Outcome of studies considered to present the strongest evidence Interrupted time series for A: Coello et al[25] B: Cosseron Zerbib et al[26] C: Duckworth et al[28] D: Faoagli et al[31] E: Farrington et al[32] F: Harbath et al.[35][36] Table 3 gives explanatory text. Asterisks indicate phases with most intensive isolation policies. In D and E isolation policies in both phases were similar (isolation wards), but in the second phase the capacities of the isolation wards were exceeded in both cases, and the overflow was cohorted or isolated in single rooms

. . . .

. . . .

. . . .

. . . .

. . . .

. . . .

. . . .

. . . .

. . . .

. . . .

. . . .

. . . .

. . . .

. . . .

. . . .

. . . .

. . . .

. . . .

. . . .

. . . .

Question 4

Data from the paper 'Isolation measures in the hospital management of methicillin resistant *Staphylococcus aureus* (MRSA): systematic review of the literature' (with copyright permission from *British Medical Journal* 2004; 329: 533–539) are given in reference material 1.1b and 1.1c.

1 Describe the problems associated with data quality in systematic reviews

2 With reference to table 3 (reference material 1.1b), comment on the studies included

3 With regard to your brief to implement an evidence-based strategy to reduce MRSA transmission in your local community hospital, what recommendations could you make from this evidence?

. . . .

. . . .

. . . .

. . . .

. . . .

. . . .

. . . .

. . . .

. . . .

. . . .

. . . .

. . . .

. . . .

. . . .

. . . .

. . . .

Question 5

One of your partners announces that he wishes to become a GPwSI in ENT. What issues does this raise?

. . . .

. . . .

. . . .

. . . .

. . . .

. . . .

. . . .

. . . .

. . . .

. . . .

. . . .

. . . .

. . . .

. . . .

. . . .

. . . .

. . . .

. . . .

. . . .

. . . .

. . . .

. . . .

. . . .

Question 6

Your next patient is a 58-year-old man who has had progressive weakness in his right leg. His EMG results have come back showing he has motor neurone disease. What issues would you aim to cover in the consultation?

. . . .

. . . .

. . . .

. . . .

. . . .

. . . .

. . . .

. . . .

. . . .

. . . .

. . . .

. . . .

. . . .

. . . .

. . . .

. . . .

. . . .

. . . .

. . . .

. . . .

. . . .

. . . .

. . . .

. . . .

Question 7

Please read the extract from 'Efficacy and safety of naltrexone and acamprosate in the treatment of alcohol dependence: a systematic review' (*Addiction* 2004; 99: 811–828, (*Bandolier* 126:3) given in reference material 1.2a and answer the questions below.

1   Comment on the style of data presentation chosen by the authors in Figure 1 of reference material 1.2b

2   What is your interpretation of the data in Figure 1?

3   What is your interpretation of the data in Figure 2 of reference material 1.2b?

4   With regard to the data in Table 1 of reference material 1.2c, comment on the statement that 'Naltrexone is a safe and effective adjunct to the treatment of alcohol dependence'

Reference material 1.2a

Systematic review

The review sought randomised studies of full, published papers comparing acamprosate or naltrexone with placebo or other control without medication. Studies had to be longer than two weeks. The period covered in searching four electronic databases was 1990–end 2002.

Results

Acamprosate

For acamprosate there were 13 placebo-controlled trials with about 4000 subjects. Twelve were conducted in an ambulatory setting and were included in the review. All used standard definitions of alcohol dependence and all subjects had undergone a previous detoxification process. Most were double blind, and all had adequate quality scores. All but one reported an intention-to-treat result. Duration was three to 24 months, with most being six to 12 months. Most were definitely funded by the manufacturer of acamprosate; for four no information on funding source was available. The dose of acamprosate was most often set by body weight, being about 2000 mg daily in those over 60 kg, and 1300 mg a day in those below 60 kg.

Abstinence rates (percentage of patients completing the study without ingesting alcohol) varied (Figure 1), but with acamprosate were consistently higher than placebo. The overall abstinence rate was 23% with acamprosate and 15% with placebo, giving a number needed to treat to generate one more abstinent patient of 12 (95% CI 9 to 17; Table 1).

Acamprosate also had a small but significant increase in treatment compliance (Table 1). Gastrointestinal adverse events were higher with acamprosate (17% versus 11% with placebo, producing an NNH of 17; 12 to 27). Adverse event withdrawals were low, and not significantly higher with acamprosate than with placebo.

Naltrexone

For naltrexone there were 19 trials, of which 12 were randomised and double blind, and from which information was taken; all had adequate quality scores. Information was available from over 2000 subjects. One other (large) study was double-blind, but did not specify that it was randomised.

Studies used standard definitions of alcohol dependence, with subjects having undergone a previous detoxification. All were in an ambulatory setting. Duration was three to 18 months, with most studies of three or six months. Most were funded from charitable or government sources, with six funded in whole or part by a manufacturer. The dose of naltrexone was generally 50 mg daily.

There was no consistent reduction in abstinence rate with naltrexone. The abstinence rate with naltrexone of 35% was not significantly higher than the 30% with placebo (Table 1). There was a significant reduction in relapse rate to 37% with naltrexone compared with 48% with placebo (Figure 2), with an NNT of 10 (7 to 16).

Naltrexone produced a higher rate of gastrointestinal adverse events than placebo, with an NNH of 13 (9 to 21; Table 1). It also produced a higher rate of neuropsychiatric adverse events, with an NNH of 19 (11 to 73), but not serious neuropsychiatric adverse events. Adverse event discontinuation was significantly higher with naltrexone, with an NNH of 15 (11 to 22).

Reference material 1.2b

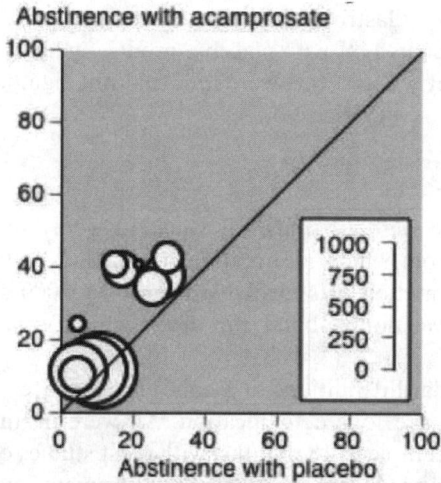

Figure 1

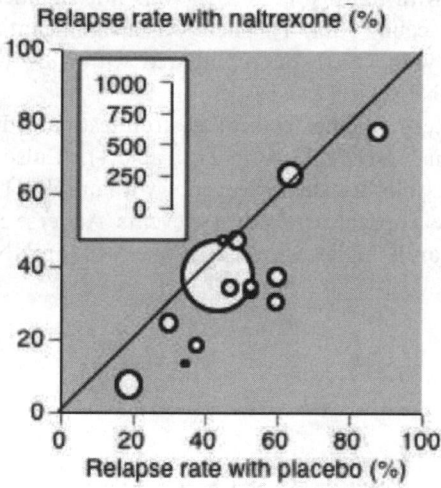

Figure 2

Reference material 1.2c

Table 1 Outcomes for benefit and adverse events with acamprosate and naltrexone compared with placebo in randomised trials

Outcome	Number of trials	Patients	Event rate (%) with		Relative benefit/risk (95% CI)	NNT/NNH (95% CI)
			Treatment	Placebo		
Acamprosate						
Abstinence	11	3322	23	15	1.6 (1.4 to 1.9)	12 (9 to 17)
Compliance	12	3959	53	47	1.1 (1.05 to 1.2)	18 (12 to 43)
Gastrointestinal adverse events	10	3425	17	11	1.5 (1.3 to 1.8)	**17 (12 to 27)**
Adverse event discontinuation	9	2697	2.8	2.2	1.3 (0.8 to 2.1)	
Naltrexone						
Abstinence	10	1077	35	30	1.2 (0.98 to 1.4)	
Relapse	14	2071	37	48	0.78 (0.71 to 0.86)	10 (7 to 16)
Gastrointestinal adverse events	17	2564	24	16	1.5 (1.3 to 1.8)	**13 (9 to 21)**
Neuropsychiatric	17	2564	43	37	1.14 (1.03 to 1.26)	**19 (11 to 73)**

NNH is **bold**

Question 8

You are called in the middle of surgery by a mother who tells you that her 12-month-old daughter who has had a cold for the last couple of days is now having a fit. Describe how you would deal with this situation.

. . . .

. . . .

. . . .

. . . .

. . . .

. . . .

. . . .

. . . .

. . . .

. . . .

. . . .

. . . .

. . . .

. . . .

. . . .

. . . .

. . . .

. . . .

. . . .

. . . .

. . . .

. . . .

Question 9

With regard to routine vaccinations, discuss recent developments in the following areas:

1   5-in-1 vaccine for babies

2   Indications for varicella vaccination and use of varicella immunoglobulin in the UK

3   Construct an algorithm for the management of a pregnant woman exposed to chicken pox

. . . .

. . . .

. . . .

. . . .

. . . .

. . . .

. . . .

. . . .

. . . .

. . . .

. . . .

. . . .

. . . .

. . . .

. . . .

. . . .

. . . .

. . . .

. . . .

. . . .

Question 10

In an effort to reduce the cost of secondary referrals, your PCT proposes devolution of budgets to practice levels with the aim of encouraging practitioners to utilise alternative referral resources. Discuss the issues raised, for and against this proposal.

. . . .

. . . .

. . . .

. . . .

. . . .

. . . .

. . . .

. . . .

. . . .

. . . .

. . . .

. . . .

. . . .

. . . .

. . . .

. . . .

. . . .

. . . .

. . . .

. . . .

. . . .

Question 11

A local solicitor specialising in negligence claims writes to your practice offering £150 commission for every patient referred to him. What issues does this raise, and how would you respond?

. . . .

. . . .

. . . .

. . . .

. . . .

. . . .

. . . .

. . . .

. . . .

. . . .

. . . .

. . . .

. . . .

. . . .

. . . .

. . . .

. . . .

. . . .

. . . .

. . . .

. . . .

. . . .

. . . .

. . . .

Question 12

It has come to your attention that your practice manager is spending increasing amounts of the working week 'working from home', the accounts are not up to date and several late reminders have arrived for unpaid bills. How would you approach the situation?

. . . .

. . . .

. . . .

. . . .

. . . .

. . . .

. . . .

. . . .

. . . .

. . . .

. . . .

. . . .

. . . .

. . . .

. . . .

. . . .

. . . .

. . . .

. . . .

. . . .

· ·

· ·

· ·

· ·

· ·

· ·

· ·

· ·

· ·

· ·

· ·

· ·

· ·

· ·

· ·

· ·

· ·

· ·

· ·

· ·

· ·

· ·

· ·

· ·

Paper 2

Question 1

A PCT audit of complaints in your locality shows that your practice received twice the average number of complaints compared with other practices. What issues does this raise?

. . . .

. . . .

. . . .

. . . .

. . . .

. . . .

. . . .

. . . .

. . . .

. . . .

. . . .

. . . .

. . . .

. . . .

. . . .

. . . .

. . . .

. . . .

Question 2

Mrs Smith, an 87-year-old widow is brought to see you by her daughter who is concerned that she may have Alzheimer's. How would you address the situation and what would be the aims of your management?

. . . .

. . . .

. . . .

. . . .

. . . .

. . . .

. . . .

. . . .

. . . .

. . . .

. . . .

. . . .

. . . .

. . . .

. . . .

. . . .

. . . .

. . . .

. . . .

. . . .

. . . .

. . . .

Question 3

Concerning patient access to primary care services, comment on the advantages and disadvantages with regard to the different stakeholders involved.

. . . .

. . . .

. . . .

. . . .

. . . .

. . . .

. . . .

. . . .

. . . .

. . . .

. . . .

. . . .

. . . .

. . . .

. . . .

. . . .

. . . .

. . . .

. . . .

. . . .

. . . .

. . . .

Question 4

Mr Smith, a 78-year-old man, presents with symptoms of parkinsonism. How would you manage the situation?

. . . .

. . . .

. . . .

. . . .

. . . .

. . . .

. . . .

. . . .

. . . .

. . . .

. . . .

. . . .

. . . .

. . . .

. . . .

. . . .

. . . .

. . . .

. . . .

. . . .

. . . .

. . . .

Question 5

MRSA is an increasing problem in all aspects of healthcare. Discuss strategies for preventing and treating infection with reference to the current literature.

. . . .

. . . .

. . . .

. . . .

. . . .

. . . .

. . . .

. . . .

. . . .

. . . .

. . . .

. . . .

. . . .

. . . .

. . . .

. . . .

. . . .

. . . .

. . . .

. . . .

. . . .

. . . .

. . . .

. . . .

Question 6

Read the extract in reference material 2.1 from the paper 'Long term donepezil treatment in 565 patients with Alzheimer's disease (AD2000): randomised double blind trial. AD2000 Collaborative Group.' (with copyright permission from *The Lancet* 2004; 363: 9427) and answer the questions below.

1   Comment on the study population, study design and outcomes

2   Comment on the relevant data under the following headings:

Patients
Carers
Society

Reference material 2.1

Summary

Background

Cholinesterase inhibitors produce small improvements in cognitive and global assessments in Alzheimer's disease. We aimed to determine whether donepezil produces worthwhile improvements in disability, dependency, behavioural and psychological symptoms, carers' psychological wellbeing, or delay in institutionalisation. If so, which patients benefit, from what dose, and for how long?

Methods

565 community-resident patients with mild to moderate Alzheimer's disease entered a 12-week run-in period in which they were randomly allocated donepezil (5 mg/day) or placebo. 486 who completed this period were rerandomised to either donepezil (5 or 10 mg/day) or placebo, with double-blind treatment continuing as long as judged appropriate. Primary endpoints were entry to institutional care and progression of disability, defined by loss of either two of four basic, or six of 11 instrumental, activities on the Bristol activities of daily living scale (BADLS). Outcome assessments were sought for all patients and analysed by logrank and multilevel models.

Findings

Cognition averaged 0.8 MMSE (mini-mental state examination) points better (95% CI 0.5–1.2; p < 0.0001) and functionality 1.0 BADLS points better (0.5–1.6; p < 0.0001) with donepezil over the first 2 years. No significant benefits were seen with donepezil compared with placebo in institutionalisation (42% *vs* 44% at 3 years; p = 0.4) or progression of disability (58% *vs* 59% at 3 years; p = 0.4). The relative risk of entering institutional care in the donepezil group compared with placebo was 0.97 (95% CI 0.72–1.30; p = 0.8); the relative risk of progression of disability or entering institutional care was 0.96 (95% CI 0.74–1.24; p = 0.7). Similarly, no significant differences were seen between donepezil and placebo in behavioural and psychological symptoms, carer psychopathology, formal care costs, unpaid caregiver time, adverse events or deaths, or between 5 mg and 10 mg donepezil.

. . . .

. . . .

. . . .

. . . .

. . . .

. . . .

. . . .

. . . .

. . . .

. . . .

. . . .

. . . .

. . . .

. . . .

. . . .

. . . .

. . . .

. . . .

Question 7

The Quality and Outcomes Framework of the new GMS contract presents many new obstacles. Discuss the likely challenges and how these can be overcome.

. . . .

. . . .

. . . .

. . . .

. . . .

. . . .

. . . .

. . . .

. . . .

. . . .

. . . .

. . . .

. . . .

. . . .

. . . .

. . . .

. . . .

. . . .

. . . .

. . . .

. . . .

. . . .

. . . .

. . . .

Question 8

A 43-year-old man with a history of chronic backache presents with a 3-day history of lumbar backache with radiation to the right leg. Discuss his management with reference to the literature.

. . . .

. . . .

. . . .

. . . .

. . . .

. . . .

. . . .

. . . .

. . . .

. . . .

. . . .

. . . .

. . . .

. . . .

. . . .

. . . .

. . . .

. . . .

. . . .

. . . .

. . . .

. . . .

. . . .

Question 9

In the capacity of team doctor to a local football team you are asked to give advice on physical conditioning and training, specifically to reduce the risk of injuries during training. In an attempt to make any advice evidence based, you research the literature and come across a paper (reference material 2.2a) entitled 'Effects of stretching before and after exercising on muscle soreness and injury: systematic review' (with copyright permission of the *British Medical Journal* 2002; 325: 468–70).

1   What problems might be encountered when conducting a systematic review of this area?

2   Comment on the data in Figure 1 of reference material 2.2b

3   Comment on the data in Figure 2 of reference material 2.2b

4   What advice would you give to your team coach as a result of reading this data?

Reference material 2.2a

Abstract

Objective To determine the effects of stretching before and after exercising on muscle soreness after exercise, risk of injury, and athletic performance
Method Systematic review
Data sources Randomised or quasi-randomised studies identified by searching Medline, Embase, CINAHL, SPORTDiscus, and PEDro,and by recursive checking of bibliographies.
Main outcome measures Muscle soreness, incidence of injury, athletic performance.
Results Five studies, all of moderate quality, reported sufficient data on the effects of stretching on muscle soreness to be included in the analysis. Outcomes seemed homogeneous. Stretching produced small and statistically non-significant reductions in muscle soreness. The pooled estimate of reduction in muscle soreness 24 hours after exercising was only 0.9 mm on a 100 mm scale (95% confidence interval −2.6 mm to 4.4 mm). Data from two studies on army recruits in military training show that muscle stretching before exercising does not produce useful reductions in injury risk (pooled hazard ratio 0.95, 0.78 to 1.16).
Conclusions Stretching before or after exercising does not confer protection from muscle soreness. Stretching before exercising does not seem to confer a practically useful reduction in the risk of injury, but

the generality of this finding needs testing. Insufficient research has been done with which to determine the effects of stretching on sporting performance.

Reference material 2.2b

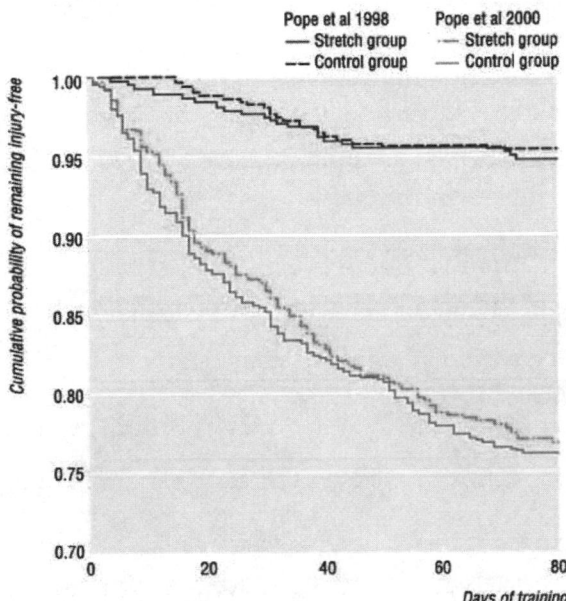

Figure 1

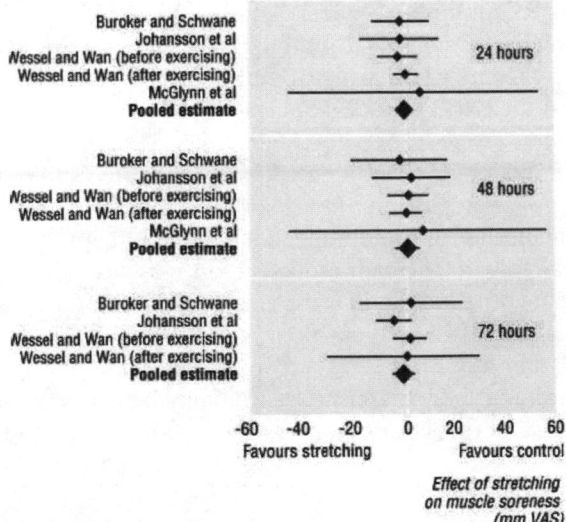

Figure 2

Question 10

As part of a prescribing review, it is apparent that prescriptions for COX 2 inhibitors are increasing rapidly. One of your partners seems to be responsible for much of this, which she justifies by arguing that money spent on drugs is more than saved on admissions for gastrointestinal bleeds. You agree to look into this.

1   How would you go about researching this topic?

2   What important considerations should be taken when assessing a new treatment for a condition?

Consider the extract in reference material 2.3 from the paper 'Comparison of lumiracoxib with naproxen and ibuprofen in the Therapeutic Arthritis Research and Gastrointestinal Event Trial (TARGET), reduction in ulcer complications: randomised controlled trial' (with copyright permission from *The Lancet* 2004; 364: 665–674). With regard to the results, calculate the following data:

3   Relative risk reduction for lumiracoxib vs NSAIDs in patients not taking aspirin

4   Absolute risk reduction for lumiracoxib vs NSAIDs in patients not taking aspirin

5   Number needed to treat with lumiracoxib instead of NSAID to prevent one case of complications, in patients not taking aspirin

6   Number needed to harm for patients taking NSAIDs without aspirin

7   Assuming that lumiracoxib costs £15 per patient per month, while conventional NSAIDs cost £3 per month, comment on the suggestion that COX 2s offer significant overall savings when cost of treating gastrointestinal complications is considered.

Reference material 2.3

Summary

Background

Cyclo-oxygenase 2 (COX2)-selective inhibitors should reduce ulcer complications compared with non-selective non-steroidal anti-inflammatory drugs, but evidence is limited, and the possibility that these inhibitors increase cardiovascular events has been raised. The Therapeutic Arthritis Research and Gastrointestinal Event Trial (TARGET) aimed to assess gastrointestinal and cardiovascular safety of the COX2 inhibitor lumiracoxib compared with two non-steroidal anti-inflammatory drugs, naproxen and ibuprofen.

Methods

18 325 patients age 50 years or older with osteoarthritis were randomised to lumiracoxib 400 mg once daily (n = 9156), naproxen 500 mg twice daily (4754), or ibuprofen 800 mg three times daily (4415) for 52 weeks, in two substudies of identical design (lumiracoxib vs ibuprofen or naproxen). Randomisation was stratified for low-dose aspirin use and age. The primary endpoint was the difference in time-to event distribution of upper gastrointestinal ulcer complications (bleeding, perforation, or obstruction); analysis was by modified intention to treat. The principal measure of adverse cardiovascular events was the Antiplatelet Trialists' Collaboration endpoint (myocardial infarction, stroke, or cardiovascular death); this analysis was intention to treat.

Findings

81 (0.44%) patients did not start treatment and 7120 (39%) did not complete the study. In patients not taking aspirin, the cumulative 1-year incidence of ulcer complications was 1.09% (95% CI 0.82–1.36) with non-steroidal anti-inflammatory drugs (64 events) versus 0.25% (95% CI 0.12–0.39) with lumiracoxib (14 events; hazard ratio 0.21 [95% CI 0.12–0.37], $p < 0.0001$). Reductions in ulcer complications were also significant in the overall population (0.34 [0.22–0.52], $p < 0.0001$) but not in those taking aspirin (0.79 [0.40–1.55], $p = 0.4876$). In the overall population, 0.55% (50/9127) of those on non-steroidal anti-inflammatory drugs and 0.65% (59/9117) of those on lumiracoxib reached the cardiovascular endpoint (1.14 [0.78–1.66], $p = 0.5074$).

Interpretation

Lumiracoxib showed a three to four-fold reduction in ulcer complications compared with non-steroidal anti-inflammatory drugs without an increase in the rate of serious cardiovascular events, suggesting that lumiracoxib is an appropriate treatment for patients with osteoarthritis.

....
....
....
....
....
....
....
....
....
....
....
....
....
....
....
....
....
....
....
....
....
....
....
....
....
....
....
....
....

Question 11

Your next patient is a 33-year-old man who works in a local factory. He tells you he had diarrhoea for three days, which has now settled, but that he needs a sick note for work. How would you approach the situation?

. . . .

. . . .

. . . .

. . . .

. . . .

. . . .

. . . .

. . . .

. . . .

. . . .

. . . .

. . . .

. . . .

. . . .

. . . .

. . . .

. . . .

. . . .

. . . .

. . . .

. . . .

. . . .

Question 12

You are interrupted in the middle of surgery by one of your nurses who has been doing the baby clinic. She has discovered that the last patient, a 18-month-old girl, received a meningitis C vaccination instead of MMR. What issues does this raise and how would you react?

. . . .

. . . .

. . . .

. . . .

. . . .

. . . .

. . . .

. . . .

. . . .

. . . .

. . . .

. . . .

. . . .

. . . .

. . . .

. . . .

. . . .

. . . .

. . . .

. . . .

. . . .

. . . .

Paper 3

Question 1

See reference material 3.1a, part of a paper entitled
'Meta-analysis of increased dose of inhaled steroid or addition
of salmeterol in symptomatic asthma (MIASMA)' (with
copyright permission from *British Medical Journal* 2000; 320:
1368–1373).

1 Comment on the outcome measures used

2 Comment on the methods for identifying suitable studies

3 Comment on the studies included

4 Comment on the results shown in Table 5 of reference material
3.1b

5 Comment on the applicability of these results to clinical
practice

Reference material 3.1a

Objective To examine the benefits of adding salmeterol compared
with increasing dose of inhaled corticosteroids.
Design Systematic review of randomised, double blind clinical trials.
Independent data extraction and validation with summary data from
study reports and manuscripts. Fixed and random effects analyses.
Setting EMBASE, Medline, and GlaxoWellcome internal clinical
study registers.
Main outcome measures Efficacy and exacerbations.

Methods

Searches

We searched EMBASE, Medline, and GlaxoWellcome databases before
the analysis started in January 1998. All publications and abstracts from
1985 onwards in all languages were considered. In a further search in
September 1999 we identified no additional studies that fulfilled the search
criteria. Study search and selection was conducted by SS.

Selection

Criteria for selection of studies for inclusion in the review were randomised controlled trials; direct comparison between addition of salmeterol to current dose of inhaled steroid and increased (at least doubling) dose of current inhaled steroid for a minimum of 12 weeks; and adults or adolescents (age 12 years or over) with symptomatic asthma on current dose of inhaled steroids.

Quality assessment

All included studies were sponsored by GlaxoWellcome and all met companywide minimum quality thresholds. All were randomised by using PACT (patient allocation for clinical trials), an in-house, computer-based randomisation package validated by the Food and Drug Administration. In all studies, maintenance of the treatment blind was carefully managed with adherence to in-house standard operating procedures. In all studies, treatment packs were supplied numbered in non-identifiable packaging and were dispensed by investigators to the next sequential patient to be randomised in the trial. All studies were conducted according to good clinical practice, and all had received ethical approval. In all studies, appropriate statistical methods were used for summarising and comparing treatments, and methods for handling missing data were preplanned.

Data abstraction

Data abstraction was based on reported summary statistics (means, SD and SE, proportions) for the intention to treat population. Two independent co-workers extracted data from study reports and manuscripts, and their results were compared. Discrepancies were resolved by consensus. Severity of exacerbation was not reported in all studies, and so individual patient datasets were sought and obtained in all but two studies. Severity of exacerbation was assessed independently by two coworkers, without knowledge of treatment allocation or results, who applied the following criteria: severe – requiring oral steroids or admission to hospital; moderate – requiring an increase in inhaled steroid medication; mild – requiring an increase in use of rescue medication.

Quantitative data synthesis

For all measures, treatments were compared each month and for months one to six (when available), with primary interest in the comparisons at three and six months. For peak expiratory flow (recorded by patients twice daily, morning and evening, on diary cards) and forced expiratory volume in one second (FEV1) (recorded at clinic visits) the measure of effect was the difference in means. Previous experience with these measures provided assurance that they have approximately normal distributions. We used reported treatment means or medians for the week or month (as reported) immediately before the next assessment, with previous experience again suggesting approximate normality. For symptoms and use of rescue medication (recorded by the patients on their diary cards) the measure was the difference in the mean percentage of days and nights without symptoms or use of rescue medication. For these measures treatment means were obtained as the mean of the patient means (or medians, as reported), which were calculated over the interval of interest. For exacerbations (recorded in case record forms) the measure was the difference in the percentage of participants with one or more exacerbations.

The primary method of combining results was by using a fixed effect model weighting according to inverse study variance. Random effects estimators were also calculated to provide an assessment of the degree of heterogeneity.[4] Evidence for statistical heterogeneity was formally tested and the potential for publication bias assessed by funnel plot.[7] All analyses were conducted with SAS v6.12.

Reference material 3.1b

Table 5 Numbers (%) of participants with one or more exacerbations of asthma according to severity and difference (95% confidence interval) between treatment with salmeterol and increased dose of inhaled steroid

Reference	Any (mild, moderate, or severe) exacerbation			Moderate or severe exacerbation		
	Salmeterol	Inhaled steroid	Difference	Salmeterol	Inhaled steroid	Difference
Greening[2]	78/220 (35)	68/206 (33)	−2.45 (−11.46 to 6.57)	19/220 (9)	18/206 (9)	0.10 (−5.25 to 5.45)
Ind[8]	60/171 (35)	60/165 (36)	1.28 (−8.97 to 11.53)	47/171 (27)	51/165 (31)	3.42 (−6.30 to 13.15)
Woolcock[9]	49/243 (20)	50/251 (20)	−0.24 (−7.31 to 6.82)	40/243 (16)	42/251 (17)	0.27 (−6.29 to 6.84)
Kelsen[10]	37/239 (15)	42/244 (17)	1.73 (−4.86 to 8.33)	18/239 (8)	26/244 (11)	3.12 (−1.99 to 8.24)
Murray[11]	40/260 (15)	44/254 (17)	1.94 (−4.46 to 8.33)	19/260 (11)	31/254 (12)	1.05 (−4.50 to 6.61)
Kalberg[12]	20/246 (8)	32/242 (13)	5.09 (−0.37 to 10.56)	15/246 (6)	27/242 (11)	5.06 (0.09 to 10.03)
Condemi[13]	21/221 (10)	31/216 (14)	4.85 (−1.22 to 10.92)	19/221 (9)	26/216 (12)	3.44 (−2.26 to 9.14)
Van Noord[14]	0/30	2/30 (7)	6.67 (−3.33 to 16.67)	NA	NA	NM
Van Noord[14]	15/109 (14)	13/105 (12)	−1.38 (−10.41 to 7.65)	NA	NA	NM
Vermetten[15]	9/113 (8)	17/120 (14)	6.20 (−1.79 to 14.19)	NA	NA	NM
Pooled results						
Fixed effect			2.73 (0.43 to 5.04)			2.42 (0.24 to 4.60)
Random effects			2.73 (0.43 to 5.04)			2.42 (0.24 to 4.60)
Heterogeneity statistic; df (P value)			5.477; 9 (0.79)			2.687; 6 (0.85)

NA Not applicable: study treatment duration only three months. NM Not measured or available for this study.

Question 2

An 18-year-old model comes to you complaining of a 3-month history of amenorrhoea. Outline your management.

. . . .

. . . .

. . . .

. . . .

. . . .

. . . .

. . . .

. . . .

. . . .

. . . .

. . . .

. . . .

. . . .

. . . .

. . . .

. . . .

. . . .

. . . .

. . . .

. . . .

. . . .

. . . .

. . . .

. . . .

Question 3

The father of an 8-year-old girl requests that you record and investigate his concerns that his estranged wife may have Munchausen's-by-proxy. What are the implications of this?

. . . .

. . . .

. . . .

. . . .

. . . .

. . . .

. . . .

. . . .

. . . .

. . . .

. . . .

. . . .

. . . .

. . . .

. . . .

. . . .

. . . .

. . . .

. . . .

. . . .

. . . .

Question 4

Mrs Bhatia is having hospital-initiated infertility treatment and attends for a repeat script. You note you wrongly prescribed her clomipramine last time instead of clomiphene. What issues does this raise?

. . . .

. . . .

. . . .

. . . .

. . . .

. . . .

. . . .

. . . .

. . . .

. . . .

. . . .

. . . .

. . . .

. . . .

. . . .

. . . .

. . . .

. . . .

. . . .

. . . .

. . . .

. . . .

Question 5

Discuss the management of the following ENT conditions, with reference to the literature:

1   Bell's palsy
2   Benign paroxysmal positional vertigo

. . . .
. . . .
. . . .
. . . .
. . . .
. . . .
. . . .
. . . .
. . . .
. . . .
. . . .
. . . .
. . . .
. . . .
. . . .
. . . .
. . . .
. . . .
. . . .
. . . .
. . . .
. . . .
. . . .
. . . .

Question 6

Your practice is considering setting up a sleep clinic for parents of children with sleep problems. Read reference material 3.2a, an abstract from the paper entitled 'Randomised controlled trial of behavioural infant sleep intervention to improve infant sleep and maternal mood' (with copyright permission from *British Medical Journal* 2002;324: 1062–1065).

1   Comment on the strengths and weaknesses of the methodology

2   Comment on the results shown in reference material 3.2b

Reference material 3.2a

Methods

Participants

This randomised controlled trial was nested within a larger survey. Between May 1998 and April 1999 all mothers attending routine screening sessions for infant hearing at maternal and child health centres in three local government areas in suburban Melbourne, Australia, were invited to complete a survey about their infant's sleep and their own wellbeing (94% response rate). About 80% of children attend these free screening sessions, which are offered to all infants aged 7–9 months.

Survey mothers were eligible for the trial if they reported a problem with their infant's sleep and at least one of the following over the preceding two weeks: waking on more than five nights a week, waking more than three times a night, taking more than 30 minutes to fall asleep, or requiring parental presence to fall asleep. We excluded mothers with insufficient English to complete questionnaires, who were receiving treatment for postnatal depression, or who reported thoughts of self harm and infants with a major medical or developmental problem and those already receiving help for their sleep problem.

Intervention

Mothers in the intervention group attended three private consultations, held fortnightly at their local maternal and child health centre. Sleep management plans were tailored towards individual families. As well as discussing normal sleep cycles, parents were taught that settling after night waking is a learned behaviour that can be modified, infants need to be taught to fall asleep independently, factors reinforcing the sleep problem can be eliminated with appropriate behavioural interventions (see below), an infant's cry may be for more than one reason, and a bedtime routine and consistent daytime naps are desirable.

The main intervention was controlled crying, whereby parents responded to their infant's cry at increasing time intervals, allowing the infant to fall asleep by itself. A few parents chose 'camping out,' whereby they sat with their infant until the infant fell asleep and gradually removed their presence over a period of three weeks. Overnight feeding that contributed to night waking was managed by reducing over seven to 10 days the volume of milk given or time taken to feed. When a dummy was causing problems (needing a parent to find and replace it), parents removed it or attached it to the infant's clothing overnight.

Mothers in the intervention group also received a sleep management plan, information about the development and management of sleep problems, and the same information about normal sleep patterns as the control group. They were asked to maintain daily sleep diaries until the first follow up questionnaire.

Control group

Mothers in the control group were mailed a single sheet describing normal sleep patterns in infants aged 6 to 12 months based on Australian normative data. This sheet did not include advice on how to manage infant sleep problems.

Process

Mothers were randomised to the intervention or control group within two strata ('depressed' and 'not depressed'). Masking occurred at three points (randomisation, data collection, and analysis). Allocation sequences were concealed from researchers and participants until allocation was complete.

We measured outcomes at two months and four months after randomisation by mailed questionnaires. The primary outcomes were maternal report of an infant sleep problem (yes or no) and symptoms of depression measured by the Edinburgh postnatal depression scale with cut off scores of > 12 and $\geqslant 10$.

Analysis

We calculated that we would need a sample of 140 women to have an 80% chance of detecting, at a two sided 5% significance level, a three point difference between the two groups in the mean change in the depression score, with an assumed SD of 4.8 and a loss to follow up of 30%.

We carried out all analyses on an intention to treat basis. Fewer women than anticipated had scores that indicated clinical depression (13 in each group) so we dichotomised depression status at recruitment using community cut off points (depression score < 10 and $\geqslant 10$) for analyses.

We used multiple regression models controlling for baseline Edinburgh depression score and allocated group to assess the impact of controlled crying on change in depression scores and factors associated with increased depression scores at two and four months.

Reference material 3.2b

Results

Participant flow and follow up

Of the 738 mothers who completed the survey, 232 were eligible to participate and left contact details and 155 of these agreed to participate.

Sleep

At two months more infant sleep problems had resolved in the intervention group than in the control group (53/76 v 36/76, P = 0.005, table 2) and remaining sleep problems were less severe in the intervention group (P = 0.01). In the subgroup of depressed mothers, significantly fewer infants of mothers in the intervention group had a sleep problem at two months (26/33 v 13/33, P = 0.001, table 2).

At two months more control mothers than intervention mothers had sought extra help (23/76 (30%) v 9/75 (12%), $\chi^2 = 7.54$, P = 0.006) (see also bmj.com). Within the control group more mothers who sought extra help reported that their infant's sleep problem had resolved (13/23 (56%) v 23/53 (43(%), $\chi^2 = 1.11$, P = 0.30).

Maternal depression

At two months depression scores fell in both groups, with a slightly greater improvement in the intervention group (table 3). After we controlled for additional professional services, Edinburgh depression score, and allocated group with multiple regression the marginally significant fall in depression scores at two months for the intervention versus control group became significant (point estimate 1.4, 95% confidence interval 0.2 to 2.5, P = 0.02). By four months the greater fall in depression score for intervention mothers was no longer significant, even when we controlled for extra help. For the subgroup of mothers with initial depression scores $\geqslant 10$, scores fell in both groups with a significantly greater improvement in the intervention group at two and four months.

Details of information and strategies that mothers in the intervention group found helpful are given on bmj.com.

Table 2 Number of mothers whose infants' sleep problems had resolved at two and four months for whole sample and subgroups according to mother's Edinburgh depression score

	Resolved at two months			Resolved at four months		
	Intervention	Control	P value*	Intervention	Control	P value*
Whole sample	53/76	36/76	0.005	48/75	39/71	0.26
By Edinburgh score:						
≥10	26/33	13/33	0.001	21/32	14/30	0.13
<10	27/43	22/43	0.34	27/43	25/41	0.86

* χ^2 test.

Table 3 Change in Edinburgh depression scale scores between baseline and two and four months for whole sample and by depression subgroup

	Baseline to two months			Baseline to four months		
	No of women	Change (95% CI)	P* value	No of women	Change (95% CI)	P* value
Whole sample						
Intervention	76	-3.7 (-4.7 to -2.7)	0.06	75	-3.6 (-4.6 to -2.5)	0.45
Control	76	-2.5 (-3.4 to -1.7)		71	-3.0 (-4.0 to -2.1)	
By depression group:						
≥10:						
Intervention	33	-6.0 (-7.5 to -4.0)	0.01	32	-6.5 (-7.9 to -5.1)	0.04
Control	33	-3.7 (-4.9 to -2.6)		30	-4.2 (-5.9 to -2.5)	
<10:						
Intervention	43	-2.0 (-3.1 to -0.8)	0.70	43	-1.4 (-2.6 to -0.2)	0.36
Control	43	-1.6 (-2.7 to -0.5)		41	-2.1 (-3.2 to -1.1)	

* Student's t test.

Question 7

How could you improve the care of teenagers?

. . . .

. . . .

. . . .

. . . .

. . . .

. . . .

. . . .

. . . .

. . . .

. . . .

. . . .

. . . .

. . . .

. . . .

. . . .

. . . .

. . . .

. . . .

. . . .

. . . .

. . . .

. . . .

. . . .

. . . .

Question 8

Mr. Green and his wife come to see you for the result of his endoscopy. This showed an inoperable gastric carcinoma. How would you proceed, and what issues would you aim to cover?

. . . .

. . . .

. . . .

. . . .

. . . .

. . . .

. . . .

. . . .

. . . .

. . . .

. . . .

. . . .

. . . .

. . . .

. . . .

. . . .

. . . .

. . . .

. . . .

. . . .

. . . .

Question 9

Outline your strategies for dealing with difficult patients.

. . . .

. . . .

. . . .

. . . .

. . . .

. . . .

. . . .

. . . .

. . . .

. . . .

. . . .

. . . .

. . . .

. . . .

. . . .

. . . .

. . . .

. . . .

. . . .

. . . .

. . . .

. . . .

Question 10

Discuss the evidence relating to the following in the diagnosis and management of dementia:

1 Prevention
2 Assessment
3 Treatments

. . . .
. . . .
. . . .
. . . .
. . . .
. . . .
. . . .
. . . .
. . . .
. . . .
. . . .
. . . .
. . . .
. . . .
. . . .
. . . .
. . . .
. . . .
. . . .
. . . .
. . . .
. . . .

Question 11

Osteoporosis is a significant problem. For each of the three parts to the question, write the answers in columns under the headings 'Factors' and 'Comments and 'evidence':

1 Prevention of osteoporosis
2 Prevention of fracture
3 Treatment of osteoporosis

. . . .

. . . .

. . . .

. . . .

. . . .

. . . .

. . . .

. . . .

. . . .

. . . .

. . . .

. . . .

. . . .

. . . .

. . . .

. . . .

. . . .

. . . .

. . . .

. . . .

. . . .

Question 12

Read reference material 3.3a, taken from a paper entitled 'A controlled trial of sustained-release bupropion, a nicotine patch, or both for smoking cessation' (with copyright permission from *New England Journal of Medicine* 1999 340; 9: 685–692).

1 Comment on the strengths and weaknesses of the methodology

2 Comment on the data in Tables 1 and 2 of reference material 3.3b

Reference material 3.3a

Methods

Subjects, screening, and randomization

Subjects were recruited at four study sites by advertisements in the media. The first subject was enrolled in August 1995, and follow-up was completed in March 1997. Of a total of 1182 persons who were screened, 893 met the screening criteria and were enrolled: 218 in Arizona, 227 in California, 220 in Nebraska, and 228 in Wisconsin. The subjects were randomly assigned to one of four treatments with use of an unequal-cell design: 160 subjects were assigned to receive placebo, 244 to receive the nicotine patch, 244 to receive bupropion, and 245 to receive bupropion and the nicotine patch. Randomization was not balanced within sites.

The subjects were screened by means of a telephone interview and a pre-treatment session that included a physical examination, electrocardiography, and chest roentgenography. The study protocol was approved by the institutional review board at each site. All participants provided written informed consent.

To be eligible for the study, subjects had to be at least 18 years of age, to smoke at least 15 cigarettes per day, to weigh at least 45.4 kg (100 lb), to be motivated to quit smoking, and to speak English. Only one smoker per household was allowed to enroll in the study. Subjects were excluded for the following reasons: serious or unstable cardiac, renal, hypertensive, pulmonary, endocrine, or neurologic disorders, as assessed by the study-site physician; ulcers; seizure or dermatologic disorders; a current diagnosis of major depressive episode or a history of panic disorder, psychosis, bipolar disorder, or eating disorders; use of a nicotine replacement therapy within six months before study enrollment; pregnancy or lactation; abuse of alcohol or a non-nicotine-containing drug within the preceding year; use of a psychoactive drug within the week before enrollment; use of an investigational drug within the month before enrollment; prior use of bupropion; current use of other smoking-cessation treatments; and regular use of any noncigarette tobacco product.

Treatment period

The treatment period was nine weeks. Target quitting dates were set for the second week, usually day 8. Participants were assessed weekly and attended a brief (15 minutes or less) individual counseling session for smoking cessation each week. Counseling topics included motivation, identification of smoking triggers, coping responses, weight management, and use of the medications. The counsellors used a standardized treatment developed by Hurt and colleagues. The subjects also received a supportive telephone call from a counselor approximately three days after the target quitting date.

Follow-up period

Follow-up assessments and relapse-prevention counseling occurred during clinic visits 10, 12, 26, and 52 weeks after the start of the study. In addition to clinic visits, subjects received eight telephone calls from a counselor during this period, one per month in months 3, 4, and 5 and 7 to 11. All follow-up counseling was less than 10 minutes in duration per call.

Medications

Subjects in the two bupropion groups received 150-mg tablets of sustained-release bupropion (Zyban, Glaxo Wellcome), and all other subjects received identical appearing tablets. In the bupropion groups, subjects received 150 mg of bupropion in the morning and a placebo tablet in the evening on days 1, 2, and 3 of treatment; and one bupropion tablet in the morning and one in the evening on days 4 to 63. All other subjects took placebo tablets twice daily from days 1 to 63. Subjects in the nicotine-patch groups used one patch (Habitrol, Novartis Consumer Health) per day for eight weeks beginning on the quitting day (day 8). All other subjects applied a placebo patch each day for eight weeks. The patches used from weeks 2 to 7 each contained 21 mg of nicotine; those used during week 8 each contained 14 mg, and those used during week 9 each contained 7 mg.

Assessments

At base line, serum cotinine, vital signs, and exhaled carbon monoxide were determined; data on smoking history were obtained; and three questionnaires were administered. The portion of the Structured Clinical Interview for the *Diagnostic and Statistical Manual of Mental Disorders,* fourth edition (DSM-IV), concerning mood disorders was used to assess whether subjects had mood disorders. The Beck Depression Inventory assesses the severity of depression. Scores of 0 to 9 are considered to be normal, scores of 10 to 18 indicate mild-to-moderate depression, scores of 19 to 29 indicate moderate-to-severe depression, and scores of 30 to 63 indicate severe depression. The Fagerström Tolerance Questionnaire measures nicotine dependence. Scores can range from 0 to 11, with higher scores indicating more severe dependence.

During the treatment period, vital signs were assessed and the carbon monoxide content of expired air was measured. All subjects were asked to keep a daily diary for the first 12 weeks of the study that included information on smoking status, craving, and withdrawal symptoms. During the follow-up period, the Beck Depression Inventory was given, vital signs and the carbon monoxide content of expired air were measured, and self-reported smoking status was assessed.

Measures of outcome

All 893 subjects were included in analyses of the primary outcome. The primary outcome variable was the point-prevalence rate of abstinence at 6 and 12 months of follow-up. Subjects were considered to be abstinent if they reported not smoking since the preceding clinic visit and had an expired carbon monoxide concentration of 10 ppm or less. Subjects were considered to be continuously abstinent if they had not smoked after the quitting day, as confirmed by a carbon monoxide concentration of 10 ppm or less at all clinic visits during the 12-month study. Secondary outcome measures included withdrawal symptoms, body weight, and Beck Depression Inventory scores.

Statistical analysis

Chi-square and analysis of variance were used to test for base-line differences in demographic and smoking-history variables. All statistical tests were two-sided and had an alpha level of 0.05. Sample sizes were based on the results of a previous study of bupropion in which the abstinence rates at four weeks were 40 percent in the bupropion group and 24 percent in the placebo group. We estimated that 130 subjects were needed in the placebo group and 230 subjects were needed in the treatment groups for the study to have a power of 0.80 to detect such a difference at an alpha level of 0.05. All subjects who discontinued treatment early or who were lost to follow-up were classified as smokers.

Logistic-regression analysis was used to determine pairwise differences among groups in the abstinence rates. The Kaplan–Meier method was used to analyze differences in rates of continuous abstinence; homogeneity among treatments and pairwise differences were tested with the log-rank test.

Withdrawal symptoms were assessed daily with a composite score calculated as the mean of eight items in the daily diary: craving for cigarettes; restlessness; increased appetite; depressed mood; anxiety; difficulty concentrating; irritability, frustration, or anger; and difficulty sleeping (DSM-IV symptoms plus craving). The severity of each symptom was rated on a five-point scale, as absent (0), slight (1), mild (2), moderate (3), or severe (4). Repeated-measures analysis of variance was used to analyze the change in scores from base line (before smo¹ ₙ𝓰 cessation) to after smoking cessation. Group coding was used that permitted tests of the independent and interactive effects of the two pharmacotherapies. In one analysis, the changes in scores during the first six days after the quitting date were analyzed; in a second analysis, the changes in scores during each week of the eight-week period after the quitting date were analyzed. To control experiment-wise error, Tukey's studentized range test was used for pairwise group comparisons of changes in scores that were found to be significantly different; this same strategy was used to analyze body weight and Beck Depression Inventory scores. Adverse events that began or increased during the treatment phase were coded with COSTART (Coding Symbols for Thesaurus of Adverse Reaction Terms), and differences between groups were tested by Fisher's exact test.

Reference material 3.3b

Table 1 Base-line characteristics of the subjects*

Characteristic	Placebo (N = 160)	Nicotine patch (N = 244)	Bupropion (N = 244)	Nicotine patch and bupropion (N = 245)
Age (yr)	42.7 ± 10.2	44.0 ± 10.9	42.3 ± 10.2	43.9 ± 11.6
Female sex (%)	58.8	51.6	51.6	49.4
White race (%)	93.1	93.0	93.9	92.2
Weight (kg)	74.2 ± 14.6	76.9 ± 17.4	76.5 ± 16.2	76.1 ± 16.1
Education (%)				
High-school graduate or less	24.4	21.3	21.3	18.4
Some education after high school	48.1	51.2	46.3	48.6
College graduate or more	27.5	27.5	32.4	33.1
No. of cigarettes smoked daily	28.1 ± 10.6	26.5 ± 9.4	25.5 ± 8.8	26.8 ± 9.4
Years of smoking cigarettes	25.6 ± 9.9	26.8 ± 11.1	24.6 ± 10.5	26.7 ± 11.6
No. of previous attempts to quit	2.8 ± 3.0	2.7 ± 2.4	3.1 ± 4.7	2.5 ± 2.4
Expired carbon monoxide (ppm)	30.2 ± 12.2	28.3 ± 9.9	28.4 ± 11.1	28.7 ± 11.1
Serum cotinine (ng/ml)	358 ± 157	373 ± 204	357 ± 170	362 ± 165
Fagerström score†	7.5 ± 1.8	7.4 ± 1.7	7.4 ± 1.6	7.3 ± 1.8
Other smokers in household (%)	37.1	28.3	28.7	24.5
Previous use of nicotine patch (%)	36.5	38.1	36.9	34.7
Previous use of nicotine gum (%)	34.0	23.4	28.3	28.2
History of major depression (%)‡	15.6	18.0	20.9	17.6
Beck Depression Inventory score§	4.0 ± 4.4	3.9 ± 4.5	4.4 ± 5.1	3.5 ± 4.7

*Plus–minus values are means ± SD. Percentages do not all sum to 100, because of rounding.
† The range for the Fagerström Tolerance Questionnaire score is 0 to 11, with scores of 6 or greater indicating higher levels of nicotine dependence.
‡ History of major depression was assessed by the Structured Clinical Interview, for the DSM-IV. Persons meeting criteria for a current diagnosis of major depression were excluded from the study.
§ The scores on the Beck Depression Inventory can range from 0 to 63, with scores of 0 to 9 considered to be within the normal range. Scores of 10 to 18 indicate mild-to-moderate depression, scores of 19 to 29 moderate-to-severe depression, and scores of 30 or higher severe depression.

Table 2 Primary efficacy outcomes*

Outcome	Placebo (N = 160)	Nicotine patch (N = 244)	Bupropion (N = 244)	Bupropion and nicotine patch (N = 245)
No. evaluated at 6 mo	86	159	178	195
Abstinence at 6 mo – % (no.)	18.8 (30)	21.3 (52)	34.8 (85)	38.8 (95)
Odds ratio (95% CI)	–	1.2 (0.7–1.9)	2.3 (1.4–3.7)	2.7 (1.7–4.4)
P value				
For the comparison with placebo	–	0.53	<0.001	<0.001
For the comparison with patch	–	–	0.001	<0.001
For the comparison with bupropion alone	–	–	–	0.37
No. evaluated at 12 mo	82	152	169	181
Abstinence at 12 mo – % (no.)	15.6 (25)	16.4 (40)	30.3 (74)	35.5 (87)
Odds ratio (95% CI)	–	1.1 (0.6–1.8)	2.3 (1.4–3.9)	3.0 (1.8–4.9)
P value				
For the comparison with placebo	–	0.84	<0.001	<0.001
For the comparison with patch	–	–	<0.001	<0.001
For the comparison with bupropion alone	–	–	–	0.22

* Point-prevalence rates of abstinence based on biochemically confirmed (by an expired carbon monoxide concentration of ≤10 ppm) self-report of abstinence during the seven days preceding assessment of smoking status at a given time. The treatment period was nine weeks. Odds ratios were computed by logistic-regression analysis, which was used to determine pairwise differences in abstinence rates. Subjects who discontinued treatment or were lost to follow-up before a visit were classified as smokers for that visit. CI denotes confidence interval.

Paper 4

Question 1

A 45-year-old businessman consults you because he has problems getting an erection. Discuss your management.

. . . .
. . . .
. . . .
. . . .
. . . .
. . . .
. . . .
. . . .
. . . .
. . . .
. . . .
. . . .
. . . .
. . . .
. . . .
. . . .
. . . .
. . . .
. . . .

Question 2

'You can't teach an old dog new tricks.'

1 How can GPs stay up to date, and what are the risks and benefits of this?

2 Why do GPs need to keep up to date?

3 How can GPs keep up to date and what are the risks and benefits of this?

. . . .

. . . .

. . . .

. . . .

. . . .

. . . .

. . . .

. . . .

. . . .

. . . .

. . . .

. . . .

. . . .

. . . .

. . . .

. . . .

. . . .

. . . .

. . . .

. . . .

. . . .

. . . .

Question 3

A 45-year-old secretary complains of intermittent loss of sensation in her left hand. You know her father has multiple sclerosis. How would you proceed?

. . . .

. . . .

. . . .

. . . .

. . . .

. . . .

. . . .

. . . .

. . . .

. . . .

. . . .

. . . .

. . . .

. . . .

. . . .

. . . .

. . . .

. . . .

. . . .

. . . .

. . . .

. . . .

Question 4

A hostel for the homeless is to be opened in your practice area. With reference to the literature, comment on the following areas of care for such patients:

1 Barriers to care
2 Medical problems
3 Mental health needs
4 Provision of care

. . . .
. . . .
. . . .
. . . .
. . . .
. . . .
. . . .
. . . .
. . . .
. . . .
. . . .
. . . .
. . . .
. . . .
. . . .
. . . .
. . . .
. . . .
. . . .
. . . .
. . . .
. . . .

Question 5

The senior partner in your practice has the largest prescribing bill in the health authority. What are the implications of this and how would you approach the situation?

. . . .

. . . .

. . . .

. . . .

. . . .

. . . .

. . . .

. . . .

. . . .

. . . .

. . . .

. . . .

. . . .

. . . .

. . . .

. . . .

. . . .

. . . .

. . . .

. . . .

. . . .

. . . .

Question 6

A 41-year-old ex-serviceman asks for help. He complains of palpitations, nightmares and work difficulties. He smells of alcohol. His wife has seen you about relationship difficulties. Outline your approach to this problem.

. . . .

. . . .

. . . .

. . . .

. . . .

. . . .

. . . .

. . . .

. . . .

. . . .

. . . .

. . . .

. . . .

. . . .

. . . .

. . . .

. . . .

. . . .

. . . .

. . . .

. . . .

. . . .

. . . .

Question 7

Your practice is considering providing a complementary medicine service to your patients. You wish to make the decision evidence based. What are the difficulties in researching complementary therapies such as acupuncture? Comment under the headings below:

1   Study design
2   Bias and confounding
3   Results

. . . .
. . . .
. . . .
. . . .
. . . .
. . . .
. . . .
. . . .
. . . .
. . . .
. . . .
. . . .
. . . .
. . . .
. . . .
. . . .
. . . .
. . . .
. . . .
. . . .

Question 8

See reference material 4.1a, taken from the paper 'A single blind trial of reflexology for irritable bowel syndrome' (with copyright permission from *British Journal of General Practice* 2002; 52: 19–23).

1   Comment on the strengths and weaknesses of the methodology

2   Comment on the results in reference material 4.1b

Reference material 4.1a

Method

The research was conducted in a single geographical area of a city in the north of England during 1999. After full consideration of methodological debates surrounding CAM research, it was designed as a single-blind trial. Four general practices were used; all served predominantly white patients.

Tight inclusion criteria were employed. These were:
Patients currently under the care of a primary care physician following referral to a gastroenterologist;
Diagnosis of IBS in line with the Rome Criteria; and, therefore, the exclusion of other causes of symptoms.

One exclusion criterion, previous use of reflexology, was used. The purpose of this approach was threefold. First, to ensure that the IBS Classification was as standard as possible from patient to patient and that symptoms were not caused by other conditions. Secondly, to ensure that participants were chronic sufferers, thereby minimising the potential for spontaneous symptom remission or for symptom reduction owing to increased attention alone. Thirdly, the exclusion criterion was employed to ensure that patients would be unable to distinguish between treatment and control groups. Written consent from participants, and ethical approval from a Local Ethics Committee, were sought and received.

Participants, identified via a notes search, were initially contacted by their GP and then by the researcher. Ninety per cent of those sent full details agreed to participate. All were currently under the care of their GP following secondary care referral.

Patients were randomised to one of two groups:

Reflexology group. Treatment consisted of six (four weekly and two fortnightly) 30-minute sessions conducted as close as possible to 'normal' practice.

Indistinguishable control group. As benefits of CAM are frequently dismissed as the result of increased contact alone, the main aim was to control for that contact. This group were exposed to exactly the same number of contact sessions as the experimental group. Sessions were carried out in exactly the same way, following the same procedures, with the single exception that a nonreflexology foot massage was given (a massage that did not include the application of pressure on key points of the feet that is characteristic of reflexology). According to reflexology theory this should have no curative effect as no stimulation of healing has occurred.

All sessions were conducted in the participants' surgery. 'Holistic' features of a standard consultation, such as lifestyle advice, were excluded from the procedure. This was because it can be argued that the fundamental validity of reflexology rests on the extent to which its specific form of foot massage produces an impact a discernible change unrelated either to the process of consulting or to behavioural change. The study's lead reflexologist was consulted throughout to minimise grounds for the *post hoc* rejection of findings by advocates of reflexology on the basis of the inappropriateness or artificiality of project design. A written code of conduct, refined during pilot work with two people from outside of the trial, was followed to maximise procedural rigour.

Randomisation by alternation was used. Participants were recruited practice by practice since, given the small numbers involved in each practice, full randomisation in these small blocks would have been impractical.

A Health Assessment Sheet, similar to those used successfully in other IBS trials, was used to provide a quick and easy means for participants to record symptom intensity. The defining symptoms of IBS – abdominal pain and constipation/diarrhoea, plus bloatedness/abdominal distension, were assessed daily on a five-point (0 to 4) scale. The forms were completed by all participants for two weeks before the first session (details of sessions below), throughout the intervention, for two weeks after, and again for two weeks at follow-up three months after the final session. Results are based on a comparison of symptoms at baseline: end of Week 2 (prior to the first session), and outcome: Week 10 (after the last session). Follow-up data were based on a comparison of symptom intensity at baseline with symptom intensity three months after the end of the intervention. There was an 80% power (aiming at 18 patients per arm), with 5% significance to detect a difference of 50% of controls and 90% of the experimental group achieving health improvement on the principal outcome measure (abdominal pain). As no published evidence existed in the area, the figures resulted from an assessment of the kind of difference that would be regarded as clinically significant (and from clinical experience might be anticipated), i.e., the kind of difference that might underpin integration into mainstream practice. Data were analysed using a Mann–Whitney U test.

Reference material 4.1b

Results

Thirty-four patients (28 female, six male, mean age = 48, age range = 19 to 72) a number larger than in much of the related work on IBS and CAM[142°] – completed the study. Symptom duration ranged from 18 months to 15 years. Baseline depression was negligible (mean = 3.6, Hospital Anxiety and Depression Scale [HAD]), baseline anxiety was higher (mean = 9.6 HAD, 7 to 10 indicates mild anxiety, 11 to 14 indicates moderate anxiety). The intervention was completed by 19 participants in the reflexology group (15 at the three-month follow-up) and 15 in the control group (13 at the three-month follow-up).

There were no significant differences in baseline characteristics between the two groups (abdominal pain: reflexology – median = 1.4, interquartile range (OR) = 0.6 to 21, control – median = 0.7, IQR = 0.5 to 1.3; constipation/ diarrhoea: reflexology median = 1.9, OR = 1.2 to 2.1, control - median = 1.2, IQR = 0.3 to 1.7; bloatedness: reflexology median = 2.5, OR = 1.3 to 3.1, control – median = 2.0, OR = 1.0 to 2.2).

Fifteen participants were approached at varying stages of the trial and asked if they could confidently identify which group they belonged to. None expressed a 'confident' assessment although two offered a 'guess' and both of these guesses were correct. A reasonable degree of confidence that the blind nature of the trial was maintained can therefore be expressed.

Abdominal pain

Abdominal pain is the principal outcome measure and one of the key defining symptoms of IBS laid out in the Rome Criteria. These data show no significant difference between the impact of reflexology and control on this symptom (control – median = −0.40, OR = −0.90 to 0.00, n = 15; reflexology – median = −0.10, OR = −0.80 to 0.10, n = 19; U = 114.0, P = 0.32; Figure 2). No change in outcome was recorded at the three-month follow-up (control – median = −0.25, reflexology – median = 0.00).

Constipation/diarrhoea

This is the second variable drawn from the Rome Criteria for IBS. Again, there is no evidence of any difference between the groups (Figure 3), and on this measure very little impact was recorded at alt (control – median = −0.30, IQR = −0.80 to 0.20, n = 15; reflexology median = 0.05, IQR = −0.53 to 0.43, n = 18; U = 115.0, P = 0.47). This was confirmed at follow-up (control median = 0.00; reflexology – median = 0.10).

Bloatedness

The pattern established with the first two symptoms is repeated with bloatedness (Figure 4) (control – median = −0.40, IQR = −1.05 to −0.15, n = 13; reflexology – median = −0.10, IQR = −0.60 to 0.20, n = 17; U = 77.5, P = 0.17. Again, these results were confirmed at follow-up (control – median = −0.42; reflexology median = −0.10).

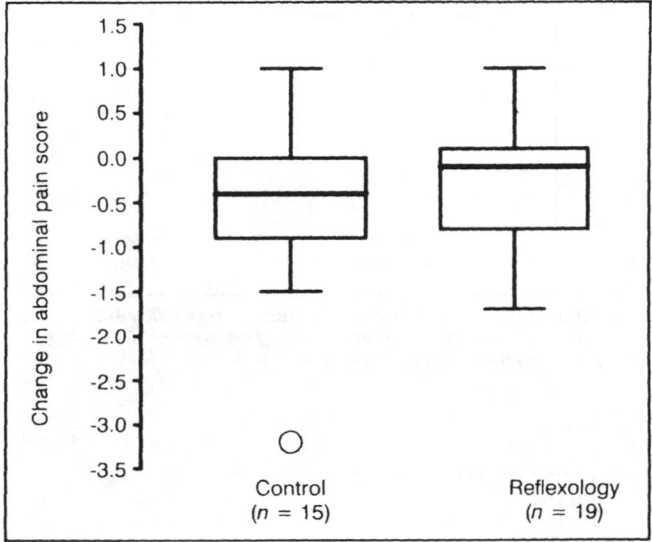

Figure 2. Change in abdominal pain score at end of intervention.
Key: ☐ *IQR;* —*median;* ⊢—⊣ *all data excluding outliers;* ○*outliers*
(> 1.5 x IQR from the edge of the box).

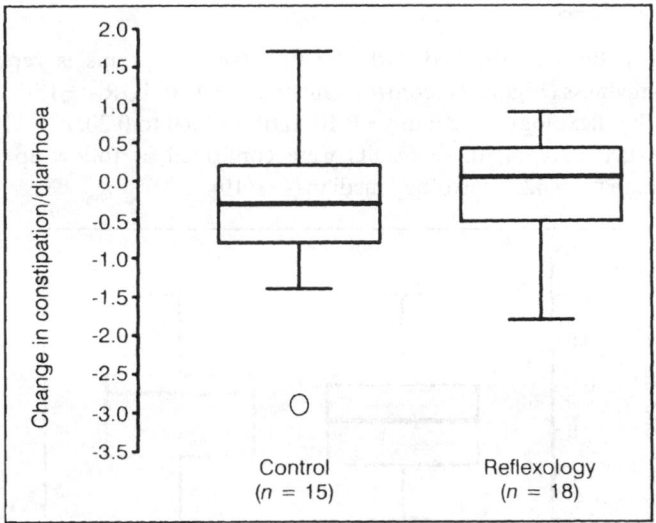

Figure 3. Change in constipation/diarrhoea at end of intervention.
Key: ☐ IQR; — median; ⊢⊣ all data excluding outliers; ○ outliers
(> 1.5 x IQR from the edge of the box).

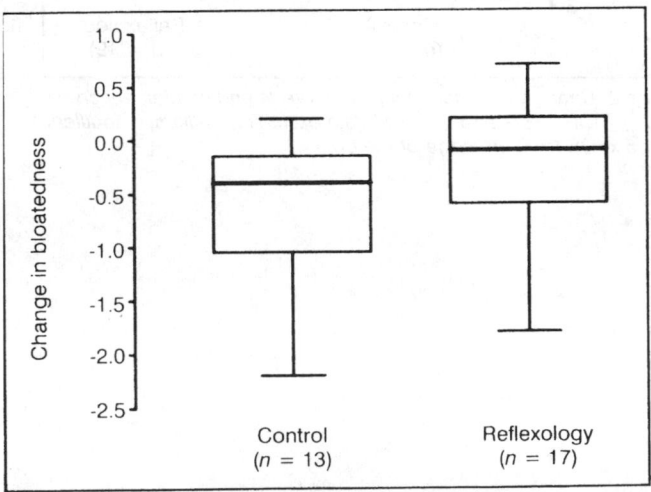

Figure 4. Change in bloatedness at end of intervention.
Key: ☐ IQR; — median; ⊢⊣ all data excluding outliers; ○ outliers
(> 1.5 x IQR from the edge of the box).

....

....

....

....

....

....

....

....

....

....

....

....

....

....

....

....

....

....

....

....

....

....

....

....

....

Question 9

Your practice is considering becoming paperless. What considerations may surround this decision?

. . . .

. . . .

. . . .

. . . .

. . . .

. . . .

. . . .

. . . .

. . . .

. . . .

. . . .

. . . .

. . . .

. . . .

. . . .

. . . .

. . . .

. . . .

. . . .

. . . .

. . . .

. . . .

Question 10

A 38-year-old woman with knee pain informs you during the consultation that her husband is clinical director of the local hospital. What considerations affect the consultation, and how would you proceed?

. . . .

. . . .

. . . .

. . . .

. . . .

. . . .

. . . .

. . . .

. . . .

. . . .

. . . .

. . . .

. . . .

. . . .

. . . .

. . . .

. . . .

. . . .

. . . .

. . . .

. . . .

. . . .

Question 11

With reference to current literature, discuss the following areas of primary care management of dyspepsia:

1 Investigations
2 Interventions

. . . .

. . . .

. . . .

. . . .

. . . .

. . . .

. . . .

. . . .

. . . .

. . . .

. . . .

. . . .

. . . .

. . . .

. . . .

. . . .

. . . .

. . . .

. . . .

. . . .

. . . .

. . . .

Question 12

'Statins: a panacea for all ills?'

Comment on this statement, with reference to current evidence.

. . . .

. . . .

. . . .

. . . .

. . . .

. . . .

. . . .

. . . .

. . . .

. . . .

. . . .

. . . .

. . . .

. . . .

. . . .

. . . .

. . . .

. . . .

. . . .

. . . .

. . . .

. . . .
. . . .
. . . .
. . . .
. . . .
. . . .
. . . .
. . . .
. . . .
. . . .
. . . .
. . . .
. . . .
. . . .
. . . .
. . . .
. . . .
. . . .
. . . .
. . . .
. . . .
. . . .
. . . .
. . . .
. . . .
. . . .
. . . .
. . . .
. . . .

Paper 5

Question 1

See reference material 5.1a, an extract from 'Survival outcome of care by specialist surgeons in breast cancer: a study of 3786 patients in the west of Scotland' (with copyright permission from the *British Medical Journal* 1996; 312: 145–148).

1 Comment on the design of the study

2 Comment on the results in table 1 (reference material 5.1b)

3 Give possible alternative explanations

Reference material 5.1a

Patients and methods

We identified all patients with breast cancer aged under 75 years whose disease was recorded in the west of Scotland cancer registry as histologically verified and who lived in a geographically defined area between 1 January 1980 and 30 June 1988 (when the United Kingdom national breast screening programme began locally).

The study population was defined by identifying the postcode sectors that formed the natural catchment areas for each of 10 hospitals concerned, which remain anonymous for reasons of confidentiality.

This procedure produced a population base of 1.5 million and 3786 histologically verified cases of breast cancer in women. We were unable to find the pathology records for only 2% of cases. Cases which were not histologically verified were excluded from the study. Of patients with breast cancer within the study area, 89% or more were treated at their local hospital. The pathology departments of all hospitals in the study area gave access to their data on tumour size and nodal involvement. Histological grade was available from only two of the 10 hospitals studied and applied to 412 patients from these.

The specialist surgeons were chosen by local perception. Over the time period of the study they each demonstrated the following indicators of specialist interest. These were setting up of a dedicated breast clinic; a defined association with pathologists and oncologists; organising and facilitating clinical trials; and maintaining a separate record of all patients with breast cancer in their care.

They kindly supplied the names of all patients in the care of their teams within the time period 1980 to mid-1988. A total of 918 patients were categorised in this way. The 2868 remaining patients were considered to have received non-specialist care. An independent scrutiny of surgeons' names on the pathology reports confirmed that the names of the patients supplied by the specialists were accurate and complete. We also confirmed that the remaining patients were indeed cared for by those categorised as non-specialists. The names of the non-specialists in the hospitals studied were not abstracted. Survival of all patients up to the end of 1993 was ascertained from death certificates provided by the registrar general (Scotland) to the cancer registration system. Information on socioeconomic status was derived for the postcode sectors included in the study area by using the Carstairs deprivation index.

We carried out an initial analysis of survival outcome with adjustment for prognostic factors – age (entered as a continuous variable), deprivation category (as three separate categories), and tumour size (as three separate categories) but not nodal involvement – using Cox's proportional hazards model. An additional analysis was carried out that included nodal involvement as a prognostic factor with the categories node negative (based on four or more nodes sampled), node negative (based on one to three nodes sampled), and node positive. This took account of concern about the comparability of nodal information for patients cared for by specialists and non-specialists. Tumour size and the state of the nodes were used in preference to conventional staging as they provide a more precise measure of prognosis for an individual patient.

Reference material 3.1b

Table 1 Survival in women with breast cancer according to whether they were treated by surgeon with specialist interest

Detail	Surgeons with specialist interest	Surgeons with no specialist interest	All patients
No of women	918	2868	3786
Percentage (SE) surviving at 5 years	67% (1.6%)	58% (0.9%)	60% (0.8%)
Percentage (SE) surviving at 10 years	49% (1.9%)	41% (1.0%)	43% (0.9%)
Relative hazard ratio (95% confidence interval) adjusted for age, deprivation, and tumour size	0.83 (0.74 to 0.92)	1.0 (baseline)	
Relative hazard ratio (95% confidence interval) adjusted for age, deprivation, tumour size, and nodal involvement	0.84 (0.75 to 0.94)	1.0 (baseline)	

. . . .
. . . .
. . . .
. . . .
. . . .
. . . .
. . . .
. . . .
. . . .
. . . .
. . . .
. . . .
. . . .
. . . .
. . . .
. . . .
. . . .
. . . .
. . . .
. . . .
. . . .
. . . .
. . . .
. . . .
. . . .
. . . .
. . . .
. . . .
. . . .

Question 2

A concerned father brings his 14-year-old son asking you to screen him for drugs. Discuss the issues this raises.

. . . .
. . . .
. . . .
. . . .
. . . .
. . . .
. . . .
. . . .
. . . .
. . . .
. . . .
. . . .
. . . .
. . . .
. . . .
. . . .
. . . .
. . . .
. . . .
. . . .
. . . .
. . . .
. . . .

Question 3

A 33-year-old man asks to be referred for a circumcision, informing you that this was suggested after a consultation over the internet for premature ejaculation. Outline your management of this consultation.

. . . .

. . . .

. . . .

. . . .

. . . .

. . . .

. . . .

. . . .

. . . .

. . . .

. . . .

. . . .

. . . .

. . . .

. . . .

. . . .

. . . .

. . . .

. . . .

. . . .

. . . .

. . . .

. . . .

. . . .

Question 4

Patients with cardiological conditions are increasingly being cared for in primary care. Discuss the latest developments with regard to the following areas:

1 Atrial fibrillation
2 Cardiac rehabilitation
3 Antiplatelet therapy for ischaemic heart disease

Question 5

A 15-year-old girl complains of problems 'down below'. What issues surround this consultation?

. . . .

. . . .

. . . .

. . . .

. . . .

. . . .

. . . .

. . . .

. . . .

. . . .

. . . .

. . . .

. . . .

. . . .

. . . .

. . . .

. . . .

. . . .

. . . .

. . . .

. . . .

Question 6

A 48-year-old woman asks for a repeat thyroxine script, started recently for weight loss by one of your partners. Her BMI is 26 and no thyroid blood tests are recorded. How do you manage this request?

. . . .

. . . .

. . . .

. . . .

. . . .

. . . .

. . . .

. . . .

. . . .

. . . .

. . . .

. . . .

. . . .

. . . .

. . . .

. . . .

. . . .

. . . .

. . . .

. . . .

. . . .

. . . .

Question 7

What are the difficulties in dealing with doctors as patients?

. . . .
. . . .
. . . .
. . . .
. . . .
. . . .
. . . .
. . . .
. . . .
. . . .
. . . .
. . . .
. . . .
. . . .
. . . .
. . . .
. . . .
. . . .
. . . .
. . . .
. . . .
. . . .
. . . .
. . . .
. . . .

Question 8

You are a member of a working party carrying out a review of community care of patients with Parkinson's disease. You are keen to make any decisions evidence based.

1   Outline how you would gather your evidence

2   Details of the methodology of one paper being discussed ('Effects of community based nurses specialising in Parkinson's disease on health outcomes and costs: randomised controlled trial', *British Medical Journal* 2002; 324: 1072–1075) are given in reference material 5.2a. (With copyright permission from the *British Medical Journal*.) Comment on the strengths and weaknesses of the study design, intervention and sampling methods

Reference material 5.2a

Methods

Recruitment

Our sampling frame included all English health authorities coterminous with local authorities in 1995 that did not already have well developed community based services of nurse specialists in Parkinson's disease. After random selection, we recruited nine health authorities (see bmj.com).

We approached all the general practices in the nine areas and asked them to identify patients with a diagnosis of Parkinson's disease from their doctor or hospital. Eligible patients were those taking one or more anti-parkinsonian drugs. They were invited to take part by letter from either their doctor or us. We excluded patients aged 17 years or less or those with severe mental illness or cognitive impairment sufficient (in the view of their doctor) to preclude valid informed consent.

Statistical power and randomisation

With an expected dropout rate of 15% in each year of the trial, we determined a total initial sample size of 1600 patients could detect a 10% change in a categorical outcome having an initial prevalence of 50%, with 80% power at the 5% significance level. Patients were randomised within practice by using block randomisation lists that reflected the randomisation ratio of the health authority area (see bmj.com).

Nurse intervention

Nine nurses were employed by the university and trained at the Nursing and

Midwifery School, University of Sheffield. They completed a course on meeting the special needs of people with Parkinson's disease and their carers. In the trial their clinical position in the community was advisory to the general practitioner rather than clinically autonomous. Each nurse was supplied with a leased car and a mobile phone and assumed areas of responsibility (box) under the guidance of a nurse manager. Their working pattern was characterised by a t' ic use study in which the nurses kept a diary of their daily work over two one-week periods. Patients in the control group were not provided with additional services until the end of the two year intervention, when they were offered one assessment from a nurse specialist.

Baseline and follow up assessments

Trained lay interviewers collected information relevant to health outcome and costs at baseline and at one and two years. Before each interview the patients were sent a questionnaire eliciting information about self-perceived health status.

Self-completed questionnaire

The questionnaire included a validated instrument for measuring the functioning and wellbeing of patients with Parkinson's disease, the PDQ-39, and the Euroqol, a health-related quality-of-life measure. The questionnaires at one and two years also included a self-perceived global health question asking patients about change in their general health over the preceding 12 months. This question is used by clinicians specialising in Parkinson's disease to gauge patient perception of changes in wellbeing between visits to hospital clinics. The five possible responses to this question were much better (score 0), better (1), same (2), worse (3), and much worse (4). Because the response in the second year depends on the response in the first year, a score was derived representing an individual's change in health over the two year period (see bmj.com). The score ranged from 0 (best) to 8 (worst).

Interviews

Face to face interviews covered three broad groups of questions: assessment of clinical outcome measures, use of health and social services, and personal characteristics. Clinical assessment included questions relating to duration and severity of disease and a test of patients' ability to put dots in a grid of 90 squares within 30 seconds (dot in square test). The Columbian rating scale was used to test patients' ability to rise from a chair with a hard seat to allow 'push off'. Adverse events such as fractures were also recorded.

Costs

Services, aids, and adaptations to the home were valued by using data compiled by the Personal Social Services Research Unit and priced at 1996 Costs; drugs were priced from the *Monthly Index of Medical Specialities* 1996 net ingredient costs. For all these elements average costs were calculated by summing the unit cost per patient, annualising where appropriate, and dividing the total by the number of patients in the study. Costs incurred by carers are not reported here. The interviews were repeated at one and two years. Follow up of mortality continued for 4 years (to 31 December 1999).

Statistical analysis

We estimated between group differences using ordinal logistic regression for progression on stand-up test, logistic regression for bone fracture, ordinary linear regression for dot in square scores and quality of life measures, and Cox regression for mortality. For each patient we calculated the changes in healthcare cost (excluding costs for carer and social security benefit) over the two years.

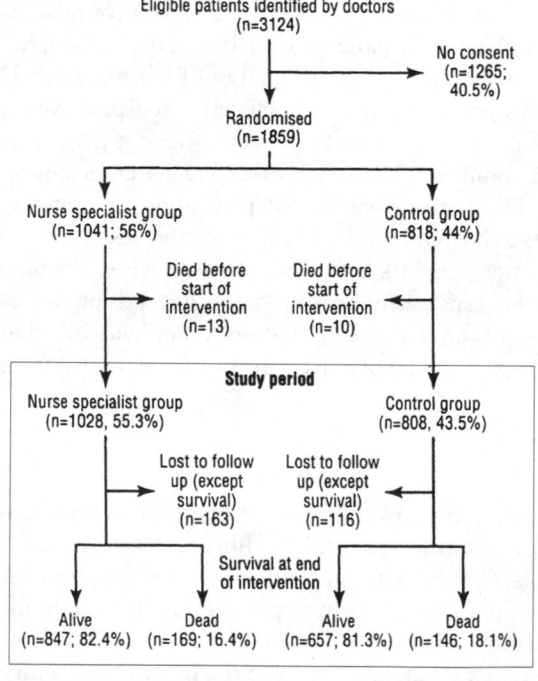

Participant flow through study

. . . .

. . . .

. . . .

. . . .

. . . .

. . . .

. . . .

. . . .

. . . .

. . . .

. . . .

. . . .

. . . .

. . . .

. . . .

. . . .

. . . .

. . . .

. . . .

. . . .

. . . .

. . . .

. . . .

. . . .

. . . .

Question 9

Extracts from the results of the paper entitled 'Effects of community-based nurses specialising in Parkinson's disease on health outcomes and costs: randomised controlled trial' (*British Medical Journal* 2002; 324: 1072–1075) are given in reference material 5.3a. (With copyright permission from *British Medical Journal*.)

1   How do the results support a decision in favour of the intervention?

2   How do the presented results support a decision against the intervention?

3   Comment on the analysis of the costs

4   Are there any other explanations for the lack of effect in the results?

Reference material 5.3a

Results

Participant flow and follow up

Of the 863 eligible practices, 438 (51%) agreed to participate and 1859 patients with Parkinson's disease were randomised (figure). No noticeable differences were observed between treatment groups at baseline (table 1). At the end of the study, patients showed a decline in health status (see bmj.com). The average self-perceived health score as assessed by the global health question was 4.89, another indicator of deterioration; unchanged self-perceived health over 2 years would score 4 on this question.

Primary outcomes

Objective measures of health

At two years' follow up the severity of Parkinson's disease, the proportion of each group sustaining a fracture, and mortality was not significantly different between the two groups (table 2).

Patient wellbeing

No differences were observed in Euroqol scores or in any dimension of the PDQ-39 at the end of the study (see bmj.com). However, when the patients were asked about change in general health in the global health question, the combined scores from years 1 and 2 differed between groups, with the nurse group doing significantly better than the control group (difference in means −0.23, 95% confidence interval −0.4 to −0.06).

Costs

The mean annual cost among the nurse group increased from £4050 in the year preceding the study to £5860 in the second year of the study and from £3480 to £5630 among the control group, the difference in mean increase between groups not being significant (table 3). The mean costs of different components of health care were also similar in each group during the second year; the provision of nurse specialist care cost £200 per patient per year.

Nurse activity

The time use study showed that the nurse specialists assessed an average of 14 patients per week, 75% at home, 14% at general practices, and 11% in hospital consultant clinics. Patients in the nurse group received on average eight assessments by the nurse per year. In a typical week the nurses made five visits to general practitioners, two to carers, and one to a consultant to discuss patient care. Apart from face-to-face contact, considerable amounts of nurse time were spent each week on administration, letter writing, telephoning patients (6 hours), and travelling (8.4 hours).

Reference material 5.3a (continued)

Table 1 Characteristics of participants at beginning of study, by treatment group. Values are numbers (percentages) unless stated otherwise

	Nurse group (n=1028)	Control group (n=808)
Sociodemographic characteristics		
Age (years):		
<70	354 (34.4)	256 (31.7)
70–77	359 (34.9)	290 (35.9)
>77	315 (30.6)	262 (32.4)
Male	588 (57.2)	456 (56.4)
Accommodation:		
Free living	916 (89.1)	716 (88.6)
Sheltered	47 (4.6)	41 (5.1)
Institution	65 (6.3)	51 (6.3)
Free living, with main carer	631 (61.4)	489 (60.5)
Manual social class	462 (44.9)	382 (47.3)
Health measures		
Years since diagnosis*:		
0–4	517 (50.3)	400 (49.5)
5–9	211 (20.5)	183 (22.6)
>9	247 (24.0)	187 (23.1)
Stand-up group†:		
1, no problems	453 (46)	344 (42.6)
2, without holding on	187 (18.2)	155 (19.2)
3, unable or had to hold on	353 (34.3)	299 (37.0)
Bone fracture in past 12 months	55 (5.4)	50 (6.2)
Mean (SD) best hand score‡	45.6 (21.7)	45.0 (21.8)
Drugs:		
Levodopa	869 (84.5)	695 (86.0)
Levodopa and anticholinergic	98 (9.5)	62 (7.7)
Levodopa and dopamine agonist	84 (8.2)	45 (5.6)
Levodopa (mg daily), median (quartiles)	300 (150, 550)	300 (150, 500)
Mean (SD) Euroqol score	0.43 (0.35)	0.43 (0.36)
Mean (SD) PDQ-39 summary score	37.9 (21.8)	38.2 (21.8)

* Missing data as some patients unaware of time since diagnosis.
† Missing data as some patients refused test.
‡ Dot in square test.

Table 2 Clinical outcomes at end of study. Values are numbers (percentages) unless stated otherwise

	Nurse group (n=696)	Control group (n=558)	Odds ratio (95% CI) (nurse v control)	P value
Stand-up group*:				
1, no problems	248 (35.6)	221 (39.6)	1.15 (0.93 to 1.42)	0.19
2, without holding on	114 (16.4)	82 (14.7)		
3, unable or had to hold on	329 (47.3)	247 (44.3)		
Bone fracture during study	92 (13.2)	62 (11.1)	1.20 (0.85 to 1.69)	0.31
Mean (SD) best hand score†	45.3 (21.2)	46.0 (21.1)	−0.70 (−3.25 to 1.84)‡	0.59
Mortality:	(n=1016)	(n=803)		
Died by 1 January 1998 (2 years)	169 (16.6)	146 (18.2)	0.91 (0.73 to 1.13)§	0.38
Died by 1 January 2000 (4 years)	353 (34.7)	307 (38.2)	0.89 (0.76 to 1.03)§	0.12

* Missing data as some patients refused test.
† Dot in square test.
‡ Regression coefficient and confidence interval from linear regression model.
§ Hazard ratio.

Table 3 NHS and local authority costs (in £000s), excluding benefits. Values are mean (maximum)

	Nurse group (n=1028)	Control group (n=808)
Year preceding study*	4.05 (55.4)	3.48 (35.0)
Year 2†	5.86 (39.1)	5.63 (33.1)
Individual mean increase†	2.54 (34.6)	2.80 (31.6)‡
Cost components in year 2†		
Nurse specialist	0.20	
Institutional cost	2.86 (20.6)	3.31 (20.6)
Respite care	0.09 (12.8)	0.08 (7.98)
Hospital cost	0.79 (17.9)	0.74 (22.3)
Primary health care	0.15 (6.34)	0.19 (6.34)
Therapy	0.10 (4.33)	0.10 (4.71)
Drugs§	0.70 (25.3)	1.12 (3.74)
Home help	0.34 (2.50)	0.30 (2.50)

* All patients entering study.
† Patients at end of study.
‡ P value 0.47 (difference −0.26, −0.98 to 0.45) (unpaired t test with unequal variances). P value and 95% confidence interval checked with 2000 bootstrapped samples.
§ Excludes apomorphine.

....
....
....
....
....
....
....
....
....
....
....
....
....
....
....
....
....
....
....
....
....
....
....
....
....
....
....

Question 10

You see a 55-year-old woman who works in a pottery with her husband. She tells you she has been seen at the walk-in centre, where she was told that she should be referred to the allergy clinic regarding a rash. What issues does this raise, and how would you proceed?

. . . .

. . . .

. . . .

. . . .

. . . .

. . . .

. . . .

. . . .

. . . .

. . . .

. . . .

. . . .

. . . .

. . . .

. . . .

. . . .

. . . .

. . . .

. . . .

. . . .

. . . .

Question 11

1 With reference to recent literature discuss the role of nurse practitioners in primary care.

2 Are nurse practitioners effective for chronic disease management?

3 Are they useful for emergency appointments?

4 Are they useful for telephone triage?

5 Are nurse minor illness clinics effective?

. . . .

. . . .

. . . .

. . . .

. . . .

. . . .

. . . .

. . . .

. . . .

. . . .

. . . .

. . . .

. . . .

. . . .

. . . .

. . . .

. . . .

. . . .

Question 12

With reference to the literature discuss recent developments in the diagnosis and treatment of coughs and colds.

. . . .

. . . .

. . . .

. . . .

. . . .

. . . .

. . . .

. . . .

. . . .

. . . .

. . . .

. . . .

. . . .

. . . .

. . . .

. . . .

. . . .

. . . .

. . . .

. . . .

. . . .

. . . .

. . . .

. . . .

. . . .

Paper 6

Question 1

You see a 31-year-old man who has a purulent urethral discharge. Outline your management.

. . . .

. . . .

. . . .

. . . .

. . . .

. . . .

. . . .

. . . .

. . . .

. . . .

. . . .

. . . .

. . . .

. . . .

. . . .

. . . .

. . . .

. . . .

. . . .

. . . .

Question 2

You are telephoned by the daughter of Mr Smith, an 81-year-old widower who lives alone. She lives in Canada and visits infrequently. She says that he is unsafe living alone and wants you to put him into a home. What issues does this raise?

. . . .

. . . .

. . . .

. . . .

. . . .

. . . .

. . . .

. . . .

. . . .

. . . .

. . . .

. . . .

. . . .

. . . .

. . . .

. . . .

. . . .

. . . .

. . . .

. . . .

. . . .

. . . .

. . . .

Question 3

A 14-year-old boy comes to see you with his parents, He has just been discharged from hospital after having an epileptic seizure. What issues would you aim to cover and what would be your management aims?

. . . .

. . . .

. . . .

. . . .

. . . .

. . . .

. . . .

. . . .

. . . .

. . . .

. . . .

. . . .

. . . .

. . . .

. . . .

. . . .

. . . .

. . . .

. . . .

. . . .

. . . .

. . . .

Question 4

You work in a busy urban practice with high deprivation scores. One of your partners announces at the practice meeting that he wants to become a trainer. What are the implications of his request?

. . . .

. . . .

. . . .

. . . .

. . . .

. . . .

. . . .

. . . .

. . . .

. . . .

. . . .

. . . .

. . . .

. . . .

. . . .

. . . .

. . . .

. . . .

. . . .

. . . .

. . . .

. . . .

. . . .

Question 5

Reducing suicide is a national priority. Discuss the available evidence relating to primary care in this area.

. . . .

. . . .

. . . .

. . . .

. . . .

. . . .

. . . .

. . . .

. . . .

. . . .

. . . .

. . . .

. . . .

. . . .

. . . .

. . . .

. . . .

. . . .

. . . .

. . . .

. . . .

. . . .

. . . .

. . . .

Question 6

What are the difficulties when dealing with patients who abuse opiate drugs?

. . . .

. . . .

. . . .

. . . .

. . . .

. . . .

. . . .

. . . .

. . . .

. . . .

. . . .

. . . .

. . . .

. . . .

. . . .

. . . .

. . . .

. . . .

. . . .

. . . .

. . . .

. . . .

. . . .

Question 7

Outline ways in which practices can improve access for disabled patients.

....
....
....
....
....
....
....
....
....
....
....
....
....
....
....
....
....
....
....
....
....
....
....
....

Question 8

What do current guidelines suggest regarding the following areas of management of hypertension:

1 **Initial assessment**
2 **Treatment**
3 **Statins/aspirin**

. . . .

. . . .

. . . .

. . . .

. . . .

. . . .

. . . .

. . . .

. . . .

. . . .

. . . .

. . . .

. . . .

. . . .

. . . .

. . . .

. . . .

. . . .

. . . .

. . . .

. . . .

Question 9

Mr Jones, who has complained of impotence since being treated for a heart attack, asks for a prescription for sildenafil (Viagra), which you have not previously prescribed. You agree to look into it and come across an article entitled 'Systematic review of randomised controlled trials of sildenafil (Viagra) in the treatment of male erectile dysfunction' (with copyright permission from *British Journal of General Practice* 2001; 51: 1004–1012; reference material 6.1a).

1   Comment on the selection process used

2   Comment on the trials identified (see Table 1 in reference material 6.1b)

3   Comment on the endpoints used

4   Comment on the results in Figure 1 in reference material 6.1c and their applicability to Mr Jones

Reference material 6.1a

Method

All published or unpublished randomised controlled trials comparing sildenafil with a placebo or alternative therapies were sought. Published studies were sought by computerised searches of electronic databases (MedLine, EMBASE, PsychLIT, Cochrane Library, National Research Register, Pharmline, PreMedline) in June 1999, using the keywords 'sildenafil' and 'Viagra'. There were no language restrictions. Internet search engines were used with the terms 'sildenafil' and 'Viagra'. In addition, a hand search was done of the *British Medical Journal, The Lancet, Journal of the American Medical Association, New England Journal of Medicine, British Journal of General Practice, Drug, Inpharma* and *Scrip* up to January 1999. A key source of information was the Food and Drug Administration (FDA) Center for Drug Evaluation and Research Joint Clinical Review for NDA-20–895 Viagra® (Sildenafil). Pfizer Ltd was contacted, as were experts in the field. References of all relevant studies were searched for further trial citations. The Science Citation Index was searched using all the studies identified.

An assessment of quality of all identified studies and data extraction was undertaken independently by two researchers, and they looked at concealment of allocation, blinding, losses to follow-up and intention-to-treat analysis. Discrepancies were resolved by discussion. Sildenafil is a new drug and all trials prior to its being licensed were sponsored by the drug company

Pfizer. Where trials were only available in abstract form, further information was requested from Pfizer.

Primary outcome was defined as sexual function, as measured by questions 3 and 4 (03 and 04) of the International Index of Erectile Function (IIEF). The IIEF is a questionnaire consisting of 15 items designed to measure sexual and erectile function (Box 1). It was specifically developed and validated to evaluate sildenafil. Question 3 asks 'Over the past four weeks, when you have attempted sexual intercourse how often were you able to penetrate (enter) your partner?' Question 4 asks 'Over the past four weeks, during sexual intercourse, how often were you able to maintain your erection after you have penetrated (entered) your partner?' Responses are rated on a five-point ordinal scale. Zero is scored when responders did not attempt intercourse.

Secondary outcomes were composed of other questions on the IIEF, the global efficacy question 'Did treatment improve your erections?', measures of penile rigidity, an event log (of attempted and successful intercourse), and a partner questionnaire.

Results were combined in a meta-analysis where appropriate, using RevMan version 3.

Reference material 6.1b

Trials Identified

[Table 1 (overleaf)]

Table 1 All Phase II and Phase III trials identified

Phase II trials to evaluate penile rigidity

Study ID, location, and date	Source of information	Study design	Duration	n	Treatment	Outcomes measured	Cause of ED in trial participants	Patient characteristics
105 USA Multi-centre 1996	FDA NDA-20-895[6]	4-period crossover 1-week washout	1 dose	54 54 53 53	Placebo Sildenafil 25 mg Sildenafil 50 mg Sildenafil 100 mg	Duration of ≥60% rigidity Duration of ≥80% rigidity	Broad aetiology (excluding spinal cord injury)	Mean age between 51–55 Mean duration of ED not reported
350 UK Single-centre 1993	FDA NDA-20-895[6]	2-period crossover 1-week washout	7 days	16 16	Placebo Sildenafil 25 mg	Duration of >60% rigidity Duration of >80% rigidity Event log	No established organic cause	Mean age not reported Mean duration of ED not reported
351 (Part 1) UK Single-centre 1994	FDA NDA-20-895[6] Boolell et al 1996[9]	4-period crossover ≥3-day washout	1 dose	12 12 12 12	Placebo Sildenafil 10 mg Sildenafil 25 mg Sildenafil 50 mg	Duration of >60% rigidity Duration of >80% rigidity	No established organic cause	Mean age = 48 (range = 36–63) Mean duration of ED = 3.4 years
357 (Part 1) UK Multi-centre 1994/95	FDA NDA-20-895[6] Price DE et al 1998[21]	3-period crossover 3–10 day washout	1 dose	21 21 21	Placebo Sildenafil 25 mg Sildenafil 50 mg	Duration of >60% rigidity Duration of >80% rigidity	Diabetes	Mean age = 50 (range = 29–66) Mean duration of ED = 3 years (range = 1–14) Diabetes >5 years
358 (Part 1) UK Multi-centre 1995/96	FDA NDA-20-895[6] Maytom MC et al 1999[22]	2-period crossover 3–7 day washout	1 dose	27 27	Placebo Sildenafil 50 mg	Duration of >60% rigidity	Spinal cord injury (cord level range T6-L4/5)	Mean age = 33 (range = 21–49) Mean duration of ED = 6 years. Erectile response to vibrator
360 UK Single-centre 1995/96	Eardley et al 1997[27] (abstract) Boolell et al 1996[28] (abstract)	2-period crossover 1-week washout	1 dose	17 17	Placebo Sildenafil 50 mg	Duration of >60% rigidity	No established organic cause	Mean age = 52 (range = 36–70) Median duration of ED = 1.5 years
369 UK Single-centre 1996	FDA NDA-20-895[7]	4-period crossover ≥1-week washout	1 dose	16 16 16 16	Placebo Sildenafil 100 mg Placebo Sildenafil 100 mg	Duration of >60% rigidity 4 hours after dose Duration of >60% rigidity 2 hours after dose	No established organic cause	Mean age = 55 years Mean duration of ED = 4.5 years
166–301 1995	Pfizer study report	3-period crossover ≥3-day washout	1 dose	10 10	Placebo Sildenafil 50 mg	Duration of >60% rigidity	No established organic cause	Age range = 32–69 ED for 3 months or more

Table 1 (continued)

Study ID, location and date	Source of information	Study design	Duration	n	Treatment	Outcomes measured	Cause of ED in trial participants	Patient characteristics
Phase II and III trials with clinical outcomes								
101 USA Multi-centre 1995/96	FDA NDA-20-895[7] Leu et al 1997[15] (abstract)	Fixed dose Parallel group 2-4 week treatment-free run in	24 weeks	83 86 82 83 82	Placebo Sildenafil 5 mg Sildenafil 25 mg Sildenafil 50 mg Sildenafil 100 mg	Sexual function questionnaire Event log Partner questionnaire	Broad aetiology (excluding spinal cord injury)	Mean age = 57.6 years Mean duration of ED = 4.6 years
102 USA Multi-centre 1995/96	FDA NDA-20-895[7] Goldstein et al 1998[8] Pfizer study report	Fixed dose Parallel group 4-week treatment-free run in	24 weeks	216 102 107 107	Placebo Sildenafil 25 mg Sildenafil 50 mg Sildenafil 100 mg	IIEF Global efficacy question Quality of life questionnaire Partner questionnaire Pharmacokinetic data	Broad aetiology (excluding spinal cord injury)	Mean age = 57.6 years Mean duration of ED = 3.2 years
103 USA Multi-centre 1996	FDA NDA-20-895[7] Goldstein et al 1998[8] Pfizer study report	Variable dose Parallel group 4-week treatment-free run in	12 weeks	166 163	Placebo Sildenafil 25–100 mg	IIEF Global efficacy question Quality of life questionnaire Partner questionnaire Pharmacokinetic data	Broad aetiology (excluding spinal cord injury)	Mean age = 59.5 years Mean duration of ED = 4.8 years
104 USA Multi-centre 1996	FDA NDA-20-895[7] Rendell et al 1999[16] Pfizer study report	Variable dose Parallel group 4-week treatment free run in	12 weeks	132 136	Placebo Sildenafil 50–100 mg	IIEF Global efficacy question Quality of life questionnaire Partner questionnaire Pharmacokinetic data	Diabetes	Mean age = 57 years Mean duration of ED = 5.6 years Mean duration of diabetes = 12.1 years 18.7% type 1, 81.3% type 2 diabetes
106 Canada Multi-centre 1996/97	FDA NDA-20-895[7] Pfizer study report	Fixed dose Parallel group 4-week treatment-free run in	12 weeks	122 127 124 124	Placebo Sildenafil 50 mg Sildenafil 100 mg Sildenafil 200 mg	IIEF Global efficacy question Quality of life questionnaire Partner questionnaire Pharmacokinetic data	Broad aetiology (excluding spinal cord injury)	Mean age = 58 years Mean duration of ED = 5.4 years

Study / location / year	Reference	Design	Duration	N	Treatment	Outcome measures	Aetiology	Demographics
351 (Part 11) UK Single centre 1994	FDA NDA-20-895[7] Boolell et al 1996[9]	2-period crossover 7-day washout	7 days	12 12	Placebo Sildenafil 25 mg	Patient diary	No established organic cause	Mean age 48 = (range = 36-63) Mean duration of ED = 3.4 years
353 Europe Multi-centre 1994/95	FDA NDA-20-895[7] Dinsmore et al 1996[17] (abstract)	Fixed dose Parallel group 2-week treatment-free run in	4 weeks	95 90 85 81	Placebo Sildenafil 10 mg Sildenafil 25 mg Sildenafil 50 mg	Sexual function questionnaire Global efficacy question Event log	No established organic cause	Mean age = 53 years Mean duration of ED = 4.5 years
355 UK Multi-centre 1994/95	FDA NDA-20-895[7] Eardley et al 1996[18] (abstract)	Variable dose crossover 3-week treatment-free run in	4 weeks X 2 no washout	43 44	Placebo Sildenafil 25-75 mg	Global efficacy question Event log	No established organic cause	Mean age = 53 years Mean duration of ED = 3 years
356 Europe Multi-centre 1994/95	FDA NDA-20-895[7] Bailey et al 1997[19] (abstract) Virag et al 1996[20] (abstract)	Variable dose Parallel group	8 weeks	106 99	Placebo Sildenafil 10-100 mg	Sexual function questionnaire Global efficacy question Event log	Broad aetiology	Mean age = 54 years Mean duration of ED = 4.9 years
357 (Part II) UK Multi-centre 1994/95	FDA NDA-20-895[7] Price et al 1998[21]	3-period crossover 3-10 day washout	10 days	21 21 21	Placebo Sildenafil 25 mg Sildenafil 50 mg	Global efficacy question Event log	Diabetes	Mean age = 50 (range = 29-66) Mean duration of ED = 3 years (range = 1-14). Diabetes > 5 years
358 (Part II) UK Multi-centre 1995/96	FDA NDA-20-895[7] Maytom MC et al 1999[22]	Fixed dose Parallel group	4 weeks	14 12	Placebo Sildenafil 50 mg	Sexual function questionnaire Global efficacy question Event log Partner questionnaire	Spinal cord injury (cord level range T6-L4/5)	Mean age = 33 (range 21-49) Mean duration of ED = 6 years. Erectile response to vibrator
359 UK Multi-centre 1995/96	FDA NDA20-895 7 Abel et al 1997[12] (abstract) Pfizer study report	Variable dose Parallel group 2-4 treatment-free run in period	12 weeks	54 57	Placebo Sildenafil 25-100 mg	IIEF Global efficacy question Event log	Broad aetiology	Mean age = 56 years Mean duration of ED = 4.5 years
361 Australia Multi-centre 1996	FDA NDA-20-895[7] Pfizer study report	Fixed dose Parallel group 2-week treatment-free run in	12 weeks	59 62 66 67	Placebo Sildenafil 50 mg Sildenafil 100 mg Sildenafil 200 mg	IIEF Global efficacy question Event log	Organic aetiology (excluding spinal cord injury)	Mean age = 57 years Mean duration of ED = 5.2 years

Table 1 (continued)

Study ID, location and date	Source of information	Study design	Duration	n	Treatment	Outcomes measured	Cause of ED in trial participants	Patient characteristics
363 Europe Multi-centre 1995196	FDA NDA-20-895[7] Cuzin et al 1997[13] (abstract) Pfizer study report	Variable dose Parallel group 4-week treatment-free run in	26 weeks	156 159	Placebo Sildenafil 25–100 mg	IIEF Global efficacy question Event log Quality of life questionnaire Partner questionnaire	Broad aetiology	Mean age = 54.5 years Mean duration = 4.8 years
364 Europe Multi-centre 1996	FDA NDA-20-895[7] Pfizer study report	Fixed dose Parallel group 4-week treatment-free run in	12 weeks	127 128 132 127	Placebo Sildenafil 25 mg Sildenafil 50 mg Sildenafil 100 mg	IIEF Global efficacy question Event log Quality of life questionnaire Partner questionnaire Pharmacokinetic data	Broad aetiology	Mean age = 55.8 years Duration of ED = 4.8 years
367 Europe & Australia Multi-centre 1996/97	FDA NDA-20-895[7] Giuliano et al 1999[14]	Variable dose crossover 4-week treatment-free run in	6 weeks X 2 separated by a 2-week washout	178 178	Placebo Sildenafil 25–100 mg	IIEF Global efficacy question Event log Quality of life questionnaire Partner questionnaire	Spinal cord injury	Mean age = 38 years Mean duration of ED = 11 years

Reference material 6.1b
Results Figure 1

Comparison: 05 Sildenafil compared with placebo
Outcome: 01 Global Efficacy Question

Study	Experiment n/N	Control n/N	Risk difference (95% CI Random)	Weight %	Risk difference (95% CI Random)
101	202/310	22/74		6.6	0.354 (0.237–0.471)
102	209/293	53/194		8.0	0.440 (0.359–0.521)
103	101/136	23/141		7.5	0.580 (0.484–0.675)
104	74/131	13/127		7.3	0.463 (0.363–0.562)
106	262/338	27/108		7.5	0.525 (0.432–0.618)
351	10/12	2/12		2.4	0.667 (0.368–0.965)
353	186/242	35/91		6.8	0.384 (0.217–0.497)
355	36/44	10/44		4.9	0.591 (0.423–0.759)
356	81/99	28/106		6.8	0.554 (0.441–0.667)
357	11/21	2/21		3.1	0.429 (0.181–0.676)
358	18/27	2/27		4.0	0.593 (0.389–0.796)
359	42/52	7/39		5.1	0.628 (0.467–0.789)
361	128/167	6/47		6.7	0.639 (0.524–0.754)
363	117/142	29/121		7.3	0.584 (0.486–0.683)
364	276/359	27/114		7.7	0.532 (0.443–0.621)
367	142/175	21/174		8.2	0.691 (0.615–0.766)
Total (95% CI)	1895/2548	307/1440		100.0	0.537 (0.484–0.589)

$\chi^2 = 49.17$ (df = 15); $Z = 19.88$

−1   0   1

Favours control   Favours treatment

Figure 1 Meta-analysis of results for global efficacy question

Question 10

With reference to the literature, discuss the evidence for and against the following areas of prostate cancer management:

1 Diagnosis
2 Treatment

· ·

· ·

· ·

· ·

· ·

· ·

· ·

· ·

· ·

· ·

· ·

· ·

· ·

· ·

· ·

· ·

· ·

· ·

· ·

· ·

· ·

Question 11

Your practice is looking at designing a protocol for the management of blood pressure in the nurse-led diabetic clinic. You wish the process to be evidence based. See reference material 6.2a, an extract from the paper 'Tight blood pressure control and risk of macrovascular and microvascular complications in type 2 diabetes: UK PDS 38' (with copyright permission from *British Medical Journal* 1998; 317: 703–713)

1   **Comment on the strengths and weaknesses of the methodology**

2   **Comment on the results shown in Figure 4 (reference material 6.2b)**

3   **Comment on the overall validity of the results**

4   **Comment on the generalisability of the results to general practice**

Reference material 6.2a

We studied hypertensive patients with type 2 diabetes who had been recruited to the UK prospective diabetes study. General practitioners were asked to refer patients aged 25–65 with newly diagnosed diabetes to 23 participating centres. A total of 5102 were recruited as they met the study's entry criterion (fasting plasma glucose concentration > 6 mmol/l on two mornings), were willing to join, and did not meet the exclusion criteria for the study. Exclusion criteria were ketonuria > 3 mmol/l; a history of myocardial infarction in the previous year; current angina or heart failure; more than one major vascular episode; serum creatinine concentration > 175 μmol/l; retinopathy requiring laser treatment; malignant hypertension; an uncorrected endocrine abnormality; an occupation which would preclude insulin treatment (such as heavy goods vehicle driver); a severe concurrent illness likely to limit life or require extensive systemic treatment; or inadequate understanding or unwillingness to enter the study. The patients were treated by diet alone for 3 months. Patients who remained hyperglycaemic (fasting plasma glucose 6.1–15.0 mmol/l) without diabetic symptoms were randomly allocated conventional blood glucose control, primarily by diet, or intensive control (aiming for a fasting plasma glucose concentration < 6.0 mmol/l) with additional sulphonylurea, insulin, or metformin treatment. Details of the protocol are published.

Of the 4297 patients recruited to the 20 centres participating in the hypertension in diabetes study, 243 had either died or were lost to follow up before the start of the hypertension study in 1987. Of the remaining 4054 patients, 1544 (38%) had hypertension, defined in 727 patients as a systolic blood pressure ⩾ 160 mm Hg and/or a diastolic blood pressure ⩾ 90 mm Hg or in 421 patients receiving antihypertensive treatment as a systolic pressure of $\geqslant$ 150 mm Hg and/or a diastolic blood pressure $\geqslant$ 85 Hg. Patients were enrolled on the basis of the mean of three blood pressure measurements taken at consecutive clinic visits. The exclusion criteria were a clinical requirement for strict blood pressure control (previous stroke, accelerated hypertension, cardiac failure, or renal failure) or β blockade (myocardial infarction in the previous year or current angina); severe vascular disease (more than one major vascular episode); a severe concurrent illness or contraindications to β blockers (asthma, intermittent claudication, foot ulcers, or amputations); pregnancy; or unwillingness to join the study. Of the 1544 hypertensive patients, 252 were excluded and 144 patients did not enter the study. A total of 1148 patients (637 men (55%) with a mean age of 56.4 (SD 8.1) years entered the hypertension in diabetes study between 1987 and 1991. Table 1 shows their characteristics at randomisation to blood pressure control policy.

Treatment protocol

Randomisation stratified for those with or without previous treatment for hypertension was performed by the coordinating centre. In all 758 patients were allocated tight control of blood pressure, aiming for a blood pressure $<$ 150/ 85 mm Hg (400 patients were given an angiotensin converting enzyme inhibitor (captopril) and 358 a β blocker (atenolol) as the main treatment); 390 patients were allocated a less tight control of blood pressure, aiming for a blood pressure $<$ 180/105 mm Hg but avoiding treatment with angiotensin converting enzyme inhibitors or β blockers. Sealed opaque envelopes were used and checked as described for the UK prospective diabetes study. The original blood pressure target of 200/105 mm Hg in the group assigned to less tight control was reduced in 1992 by the steering committee of the hypertension in diabetes study after publication of the results of studies in elderly, non-diabetic subjects during 1991–2. Randomisation produced balanced numbers of patients allocated to the various glucose and blood pressure treatment combinations for the UK prospective diabetes study and hypertension in diabetes study.

Captopril was usually started at a dose of 25 mg twice daily, increasing to 50 mg twice daily, and atenolol at a daily dose of 50 mg, increasing to 100 mg if required. Other agents were added if the control criteria were not met in the group assigned to tight control despite maximum allocated treatment or in the group assigned to less tight control without drug treatment. The suggested sequence was frusemide 20 mg daily (maximum 40 mg twice daily), slow release nifedipine 10 mg (maximum 40 mg) twice daily, methyldopa 250 mg (maximum 500 mg) twice daily, and prazosin 1 mg (maximum 5 mg) thrice daily.

Clinic visits

Patients visited study clinics every 3–4 months. At each visit plasma glucose concentration, blood pressure, and body weight were measured, and treatments to control blood pressure and blood glucose concentration were noted and adjusted if target values were not met. If treatments and target blood pressures were not in accord with the protocol, the coordinating centre sent letters about affected patients to the clinical centres requesting appropriate action. A central record of all apparent protocol deviations was maintained. Symptoms including any drug side effects and clinical events were noted. Physicians recorded hypoglycaemic episodes as minor if the patient was able to treat the symptoms unaided and as major if third party or medical intervention was necessary.

Blood pressure measurements

Blood pressure (diastolic phase 5) while the patient was sitting and had rested for at least five minutes was measured by a trained nurse with a Copal UA-251 or a Takeda UA-751 electronic auscultatory blood pressure reading machine (Andrew Stephens, Brighouse, West Yorkshire) or with a Hawksley random zero sphygmomanometer (Hawksley, Lancing, Sussex) in patients with atrial fibrillation. The first reading was discarded and the mean of the next three consecutive readings with a coefficient of variation below 15% was used in the study, with additional readings if required. Monthly quality assurance measurements have shown the mean difference between Takeda and Hawksley machines to be 1 (4) mm Hg or less.

Clinical examination

At entry to the UK prospective diabetes study and subsequently every three years all patients had a clinical examination which included retinal colour photography, ophthalmoscopy, measurement of visual acuity, assessment of peripheral and autonomic neuropathy, chest radiography, electrocardiography, and measurement of brachial and posterior tibial blood pressure using Doppler techniques. Annual direct ophthalmoscopy was also carried out. Every year a fasting blood sample was taken to measure glycated haemoglobin (haemoglobin A_{1c}), plasma creatinine concentration, and concentrations of urea, immunoreactive insulin, and insulin antibodies; random urine samples were taken for measurement of albumin concentration.

Visual acuity was measured with Snellen charts until 1989, after which ETDRS (early treatment of diabetic retinopathy study) charts were used to assess best corrected vision, with current refraction or through a pinhole. Retinal colour photographs of four standard 30° fields per eye (nasal, disc, macula, and temporal to macular fields) were taken plus stereophotographs of the macula. Repeat photography was arranged if the quality of the photograph was unsatisfactory. Retinal photographs were assessed at a central grading centre by two independent assessors for the presence or absence of diabetic retinopathy. Any fields with retinopathy were graded by two further senior independent assessors using a modified ETDRS final scale. Neuropathy was assessed clinically by knee and ankle reflexes, and by biothesiometer (Biomedical Instruments, Newbury, Ohio) readings taken from the lateral malleoli and the end of the big toe. A 12 lead electrocardiogram was recorded and given a Minnesota code, and a chest x ray film was taken for measurement of cardiac diameter.

Biochemistry

Biochemical methods have been reported previously. Urinary albumin concentration was measured by an immunoturbidimetric method with a normal reference range of 1.4 mg/l to 36.5 mg/l. Microalbuminuria has been defined as a urinary albumin concentration of $\geqslant$ 50 mg/l and clinical grade proteinuria as a urinary albumin concentration of $\geqslant$ 300 mg/l.

Clinical end points

Twenty one clinical end points were predefined in the study protocol. All available clinical information was gathered for possible end points – for example, copies of admission notes, operation records, death certificates, and necropsy reports. Copies of these, without reference to the patient's allocated or actual treatment, were formally presented to two independent physicians who allocated an appropriate code from the ninth revision of the international Classification of diseases (ICD-9) if the criteria for any particular clinical end point had been met. Any disagreement between the two assessors was discussed and the evidence reviewed. If agreement was not possible the information was submitted to a panel of two further independent assessors for final arbitration. The closing date for the study was 30 September 1997.

End points were aggregated for the main analyses. The three predefined primary outcome analyses were the time to the occurrence of (a) a first clinical end point related to diabetes (sudden death, death from hyperglycaemia or hypoglycaemia, fatal or non-fatal myocardial infarction, angina, heart failure, stroke, renal failure, amputation (of at least one digit), vitreous haemorrhage, retinal photocoagulation, blindness in one eye or cataract extraction); (b) death related to diabetes (death due to myocardial infarction, sudden death, stroke, peripheral vascular disease, renal disease, hyperglycaemia or hypoglycaemia); (c) death from all causes.

Secondary outcome analyses of four additional aggregates of clinical end points were used to assess the effect of treatments on different types of vascular disease. These were myocardial infarction (fatal or non-fatal myocardial infarction or sudden death), stroke (fatal or non-fatal stroke), amputation or death from peripheral vascular disease, and microvascular complications (retinopathy requiring photocoagulation, vitreous haemorrhage, and fatal or non-fatal renal failure).

Since a patient could in sequence have different end points, he or she could be included in more than one end point category.

Surrogate end points. Details of subclinical, surrogate variables have been published.

Statistical analysis

Analysis was on an intention to treat basis, comparing patients allocated to tight and less tight blood pressure control. Patients allocated to tight control with angiotensin converting enzyme inhibitors or β blockers were pooled in this paper for analysis. They are compared in the accompanying paper. Life table analyses were performed with log rank tests, and hazard ratios were obtained from Cox's proportional hazards models and used to estimate relative risks. Survival function estimates were calculated using the product limit (Kaplan–Meier) method. In the text relative risks are quoted as risk reductions and significance tests were two sided. For aggregate end points 95% confidence intervals are quoted, whereas for single end points 99% confidence intervals are quoted to allow for potential type 1 errors. Similarly, 99% confidence intervals were used to assess surrogate end points that were measured at triennial visits. Mean (SD), geometric mean (1 SD interval), or median (interquartile range) values are quoted for the biometric and biochemical variables, with values from Wilcoxon, t, or χ^2 tests for comparisons. Risk reductions for surrogate end points were derived from frequency tables. The overall values for blood pressure during a period were assessed for each patient as the mean during that period and for each allocation as the mean of patients with data in the allocation. Control of blood pressure was assessed in patients allocated to the two groups who had data at nine years of follow up.

Hypoglycaemia was determined from the number of patients allocated to a treatment and continuing with it who had one or more minor or major hypoglycaemic episodes each year. Urinary albumin concentration was measured in mg/l. Change in diabetic retinopathy was defined as a change of two steps (one step in both eyes or two or more steps in one eye) with a scale from the worse eye to the better eye that included retinal photocoagulation or vitreous haemorrhage as the most serious grade. Visual loss was defined as the best vision in either eye, deteriorating by three lines on an ETDRS chart. Both the UK prospective diabetes study and hypertension in diabetes study received ethical approval from the appropriate committee in each centre and conformed with the guidelines of the Declarations of Helsinki (1975 and 1983). All patients gave informed consent.

Reference material 6.2b

Clinical end point	Patients with aggregate end points		Absolute risk (events per 1000 patient years)		p value	Relative risk for tight control (95% CI)
	Tight control (n = 758)	Less tight control (n = 390)	Tight control	Less tight control		
Any diabetes related end point	259	170	50. 9	67.4	0.0046	0.76 (0.62 to 0.92)
Deaths related to diabetes	82	62	13.7	20.3	0.019	0.68 (0.49 to 0.94)
All cause mortality	134	83	22.4	27.2	0.17	0.82 (0.63 to 1.08)
Myocardial infarction	107	69	18.6	23.5	0.13	0.79 (0.59 to 1.07)
Stroke	38	34	6.5	11.6	0.013	0.56 (0.35 to 0.89)
Peripheral vascular disease	8	8	1.4	2.7	0.17	0.51 (0.19 to 1.37)
Microvascular disease	68	54	12.0	19.2	0.0092	0.63 (0.44 to 0.89)

0.1   10
Favours tight control   Favours less tight control

Figure 4 Numbers of patients who attained one or more clinical end points in aggregates representing specific types of clinical complications, with relative risks

Question 12

Your practice is attempting to shorten access times to comply with government targets. One of the areas you decide to concentrate on is frequent attenders. See reference material 6.3a, an extract from 'Psychosocial, lifestyle, and health status variables in predicting high attendance among adults' (with copyright permission from *British Journal of General Practice* 2001; 51: 987–994).

1   **Comment on the strengths and weaknesses of the methodology**

2   **Comment on the results given in Tables 2 and 4 of reference material 6.3b**

3   **Suggest possible interventions based on these results**

Reference material 6.3a

Method

Six general practices within a 30-mile radius of the administrative centre were chosen to give a range of sociodemographic and practice characteristics. A sample of 4000 households was randomly chosen, using equal numbers from the age-sex register of each practice. Patients from nursing homes and those aged over 80 years old were excluded owing to difficulty in completing the questionnaire. Patients were sent a letter explaining the project, the questionnaire, and one of three types of information leaflet/ booklet. The cohort was followed to assess the effectiveness of the leaflets (these results will be reported elsewhere). One adult per household was sampled to avoid contamination of groups. Where the random choice of participant from the age–sex register was a child (aged under 16 years, $n = 487$) an adult was asked to fill in a questionnaire for themselves, in addition to one for the child: this paper reports the adults' data. A second and third mailing were sent to patients who had not responded to the first questionnaire.

Questionnaire

Existing measures. We included items from previous studies, questions about lifestyle, and attitudes.

New measures. To limit type I error, where variables potentially addressed similar domains, exploratory factor analysis with varimax rotation was performed to identify a smaller number of 'latent' variables. Scales were developed based on a simple sum of the items which loaded strongly for each factor. 'New' measures included:

Health status (modified COOP WONCA chart questions). The chart component was omitted for ease of printing and scanning, leaving the wording unchanged. Factor analysis suggested a two-factor solution:

(a) 'physical health' – physical activity (rotated factor loading 0.50), bodily discomfort/pain (0.52), ability to work (0.65), and overall condition (0.50). A higher score represents poorer 'physical health' status. Cronbach's cx for the scale was 0.72, i.e. in the optimum range.

(b) 'social/emotional health' – emotional problems (0.69), social activities (0.53), quality of life (0.71), and overall functioning (0.62) (cx = 0.81). Questions about social support and change in condition did not load strongly onto either 'physical' or 'emotional' factors.

   The validity of the word format was compared with the original chart version sent one month later in 32 consecutive responders (Spearman's p = 0.80 for 'physical'; p = 0.79 for 'social/emotional').

Willingness to tolerate symptoms. Thirteen questions documented the number of days that people would wait before seeing the doctor for clinical scenarios (1 = less than one day; 2 = one to two days; 3 = three to seven days; 4 = eight to 14 days; 5 = over 14 days; 6 = would not contact). Factor analysis suggested a one-factor solution. Seven questions 'loaded' strongly: headache (0.62), constipation (0.67), diarrhoea and vomiting (0.62), indigestion and heartburn (0.66), cold and runny nose (0.64), 'flu with fever (0.66), sore throat and fever (0.71) (a = **0.8322**). Test-retest reliability of the scale after one month in 32 people was acceptable (p = 0.48).

'Personality'. Questions were based on Kokko's descriptions of personality types in high attenders (1 = 'very strongly agree', through to 7 = very strongly disagree'). Factor analysis suggested a three-factor solution.

(a) Factor 1 ('demedicalise') – 'the importance of the doctor making sure there is nothing seriously wrong' (0.56), 'the doctor checking things out quickly when unwell' (0.60), 'liking to find out as much as possible when unwell' (0.69), 'liking referral to specialist when possible' (0.73), 'liking tests when unwell' (0.75), 'wanting to know about side-effects' (0.55), and 'wanting the doctor to do something about it when unwell' (0.59) (a = 0.83).

(b) Factor 2 ('positive and interested') this 'loaded' questions about: 'changing health being outside my control' (0.56), 'my problems are more serious than the doctor thinks' (0.57), 'being worried when the doctor goes into details' (0.57), and 'wanting to just have the treatment without the doctor going into reasons' (0.62) (c~ = 0.69).

(c) Factor 3 ('medophile') this 'loaded' questions about: 'dislike of taking medicines and remedies' (0.51) 'and most illnesses get better without medicines' (0.50) (a = 0.58, owing to being only two items).

The question scoring meant that higher scores for the three factors reflected patients who disliked the medical process, were positive and interested in health, and positive about medicines, respectively. Other questions derived from Kokko's descriptions did not load onto the above factors – including 'repeated visits are normally needed to get the right treatment'.

Self-reported attendance. We were interested in those consulting the doctor or nurse more frequently than the average, i.e. five or more attendances a year (the top 25%, accounting for the majority [60%] of consultations). We assessed test-retest reliability of the question about self-reported attendance in the first 32 responders after one month. We also compared self-reported attendance for attendance documented in the notes in 270 consecutive responders.

Sample size (/3 = 0.2, a = 0.05 using the EPI INFO software). To detect risk factors with an odds ratio of 2 for high attendance, where the prevalence of higher attendance in patients with risk factors ranges from 10% to 90% and the prevalence of exposure ranges from 20% to 80%, 2202 responders were required (or 3146 allowing for 30% non-response).

Analysis

Data were scanned using Formic 3 software and analysis performed using SPSS and Stata for Windows software. Variables significantly associated with attendance (five or more per year) were entered in logistic regression models by forward selection, and retained if they remained significant (using the likelihood ratio test) and no evidence of significant multi-collinearity. To allow the reader to better assess the risk' associated with significant continuous variables (eg somatic symptom inventory, health anxiety) they were converted to ordinal variables: cut-offs were determined by the shape of the relationship with outcome rather than using pre-determined arbitrary cut-offs. The large sample allowed us to choose a 1% level of significance to limit type I error: a 1% level rather than the more conservative Bonferroni correction was chosen owing to close interrelation of many of the variables and collinearity of the hypotheses being tested. The adequacy of the model in predicting outcome was assessed by calculating the area under the receiver operator characteristic CR00) curve.

Reference material 6.3b

[Tables 2 and 4 (overleaf)]

Table 2 Sociodemographic, life events and practice variables associated with self-reported higher attendance at GP surgery (five or more times in past 12 months)

Variable	High attender (%)	Not a high attender (%)	Crude odds ratio (95% CI)	Adjusted odds ratio (95% CI)[a]	Likelihood ratio[b] σ^2 (P-value)
Sociodemographic					
Age (years)					
20	24/625 (4)	121/1901 (6)	1	1	6.5 (P = 0.090)
20–39	196/625 (31)	657/1901 (35)	1.50 (0.94–2.40)	1.77 (0.90–3.46)	
40–64	263/625 (42)	869/1901 (46)	1.53 (0.96–2.41)	1.28 (0.66–2.51)	
>64	142/625 (23)	254/1901 (13)	2.82 (1.74–4.57)	1.50 (0.72–3.11)	
Sex (female)	423/622 (68)	1083/1898 (57)	1.60 (1.32–1.94)	1.44 (1.11–1.87)	7.5 (P = 0.006)
No qualifications	257/593 (43)	479/1814 (26)	2.13 (1.76–2.59)	1.61 (1.25–2.07)	13.6 (P < 0.001)
Children at home	354/623 (57)	907/1869 (49)	1.40 (1.16–1.68)	1.07 (0.84–1.37)	0.3 (P = 0.586)
Ethnicity (non-white)	12/623 (2)	24/1887 (1)	1.52 (0.76–3.07)	1.42 (0.56–3.56)	0.5 (P = 0.464)
Marital status					
Single	92/628 (15)	317/1904 (17)	1	1	1.1 (P = 0.570)
Married	427/628 (68)	1333/1904 (70)	1.10 (0.85–1.43)	0.83 (0.58–1.18)	
Separated/widowed/divorced	109/628 (17)	254/1904 (13)	1.48 (1.07–2.04)	0.83 (0.53–1.30)	
Council house tenant	134/603 (22)	230/1859 (12)	2.02 (1.60–2.56)	1.32 (0.93–1.85)	2.4 (P = 0.118)
Occupation					
Paid employment	311/601 (52)	1316/1865 (71)	1	1	6.7 (P = 0.145)
Homemaker	62/601 (10)	174/1865 (9)	1.51 (1.10–2.07)	0.86 (0.56–1.31)	
Retired	170/601 (28)	298/1865 (16)	2.41 (1.93–3.02)	1.32 (0.95–1.82)	
Disabled	42/601 (7)	22/1865 (1)	8.08 (4.75–13.73)	1.83 (0.86–3.91)	
Unemployed	16/601 (3)	45/1865 (2)	1.50 (0.84–2.70)	1.58 (0.79–3.18)	
Life events					
0	233/630 (37)	836/1913 (44)	1	1	1.1 (P = 0.773)
1	224/630 (36)	617/1913 (32)	1.30 (1.05–1.61)	1.13 (0.85–1.49)	
2	110/630 (17)	302/1913 (16)	1.31 (1.01–1.70)	1.05 (0.74–1.48)	
3+	63/630 (10)	158/1913 (8)	1.43 (1.03–1.98)	1.20 (0.79–1.82)	

Practice

Practice				
1 U; A; F; C; DI	105/630 (17)	279/1913 (15)	1	1	8.3 ($P = 0.140$)
2 U; T; DI	117/630 (19)	281/1913 (15)	1.11 (0.81–1.51)	0.92 (0.60–1.39)
3 U; DI	101/630 (16)	282/1913 (15)	0.95 (0.69–1.31)	0.80 (0.52–1.23)
4 U; F; C; 1; T	110/630 (17)	330/1913 (17)	0.89 (0.65–1.21)	0.99 (0.65–1.50)
5 U; 1	103/630 (16)	335/1913 (18)	0.82 (0.60–1.12)	0.78 (0.51–1.18)
6 U/R; 1, C; F; M	94/630 (15)	406/1913 (21)	0.62 (0.45–0.84)	0.61 (0.40–0.92)

[a]Adjusted for other variables that were significantly associated with attendance. [b]Likelihood ratio test. U predominantly urban; U/R = urban rural mixed; T = teaching; A = academic (linked to university department); F = fundholding; I = inner city; DI = deprived inner city; M = market town.

Table 4 Somatic symptoms and health perception, attitude to doctors, and lifestyle variables that were significantly associated with self-reported higher attendance at the GP surgery (five or more times in past 12 months)

Variable	High attender %	Not a high attender %	Crude odds ratio (95% CI)	Adjusted odds ratio (95% CI)[a]	Likelihood ratio[b] σ^2 (P-value)
Symptom and health perception					
Medically unexplained symptoms					
0	113/630 (18)	653/1913 (34)	1	1	7.5 ($P = 0.006$)
1–2	172/630 (27)	626/1913 (33)	1.59 (1.22–2.06)	1.15 (0.81–1.62)	
3–5	181/630 (29)	430/1913 (22)	2.43 (1.87–3.17)	1.48 (1.04–2.09)	
6+	164/630 (26)	204/1913 (11)	4.65 (3.49–6.19)	1.62 (1.08–2.42)	
Health anxiety (Whitely Index)					
0	33/630 (5)	160/1913 (8)	1	1	10.9 ($P = 0.001$)
1–5	478/630 (76)	1606/1913 (84)	1.44 (0.98–2.13)	1.22 (0.71–2.10)	
6–7	63/630 (10)	100/1913 (5)	3.05 (1.87–4.98)	1.77 (0.90–3.46)	
8+	56/630 (9)	47/1913 (2)	5.78 (3.37–9.91)	2.78 (1.31–5.89)	
Perceived health					
Very good	85/610 (14)	590/1874 (31)	1	1	15.4 ($P < 0.001$)
Good	418/610 (69)	1204/1874 (64)	2.41 (1.87–3.10)	1.61 (1.12–2.33)	
Poor	107/610 (18)	80/1874 (4)	9.28 (6.42–13.42)	2.93 (1.71–5.03)	
Attitude to doctors					
Negative attitude (Negdoc scale)					
<18	190/602 (32)	478/1844 (26)	1	1	22.1 ($P < 0.001$)
18–20	214/602 (36)	622/1844 (34)	0.87 (0.69–1.09)	0.83 (0.62–1.11)	
21+	198/602 (33)	744/1844 (40)	0.67 (0.53–0.84)	0.48 (0.36–0.66)	
Often need to reattend to get right treatment (% disagreeing)	331/609 (54)	1344/1874 (72)	0.47 (0.39–0.57)	0.61 (0.47–0.78)	14.6 ($P < 0.001$)
Usually try chemist first (% agreeing)	352/612 (58)	1349/1884 (72)	0.54 (0.45–0.65)	0.61 (0.48–0.78)	15.2 ($P < 0.001$)
Lifestyle					
Alcohol (units/day)					
0	172/595 (29)	342/1822 (19)	1	1	10.1 ($P = 0.002$)
1	372/595 (63)	1200/1822 (66)	0.62 (0.50–0.77)	0.82 (0.61–1.09)	
2	36/595 (6)	176/1822 (10)	0.41 (0.27–0.61)	0.76 (0.46–1.27)	
3+	15/595 (3)	104/1822 (6)	0.29 (0.16–0.51)	0.25 (0.11–0.55)	

Sedentary (no brisk exercise)	253/610 (41)	632/1858 (34)	1.37 (1.14–1.66)	0.98 (0.76–1.27)	0.0 (P = 0.900)
Smoking					
Never	267/623 (43)	872/1884 (46)	1	1	0.2 (P = 0.892)
Ex-smoker	207/623 (33)	563/1884 (30)	1.20 (0.97–1.48)	0.93 (0.70–1.25)	
Current	149/623 (24)	449/1884 (24)	1.08 (0.86–1.36)	0.98 (0.72–1.34)	

[a]Adjusted for other variables which were significantly associated with attendance. [b]Likelihood ratio test.

. . . .
. . . .
. . . .
. . . .
. . . .
. . . .
. . . .
. . . .
. . . .
. . . .
. . . .
. . . .
. . . .
. . . .
. . . .
. . . .
. . . .
. . . .
. . . .
. . . .
. . . .
. . . .
. . . .
. . . .
. . . .
. . . .
. . . .
. . . .

Paper 7

Question 1

A local headmaster with type 2 diabetes refuses to take medication, preferring homoeopathic treatment. He refuses to attend the diabetic clinic. Bloods show a fasting blood sugar of 12, HbA1c 9.6, BP 184/102, BMI 36. How would you manage his care?

. . . .

. . . .

. . . .

. . . .

. . . .

. . . .

. . . .

. . . .

. . . .

. . . .

. . . .

. . . .

. . . .

. . . .

. . . .

. . . .

. . . .

. . . .

Question 2

Following an audit by the GP registrar it has been brought to your attention as trainer that one of the senior partners has been prescribing excessive amounts of benzodiazepines. What issues does this raise?

. . . .

. . . .

. . . .

. . . .

. . . .

. . . .

. . . .

. . . .

. . . .

. . . .

. . . .

. . . .

. . . .

. . . .

. . . .

. . . .

. . . .

. . . .

. . . .

. . . .

. . . .

. . . .

. . . .

Question 3

A 40-year-old civil engineer comes to you having been recently diagnosed with retinitis pigmentosa (autosomal dominant). He has two teenage daughters. What factors affect this consultation?

. . . .

. . . .

. . . .

. . . .

. . . .

. . . .

. . . .

. . . .

. . . .

. . . .

. . . .

. . . .

. . . .

. . . .

. . . .

. . . .

. . . .

. . . .

. . . .

. . . .

. . . .

Question 4

PCTs are increasingly looking to explain variation in referrals rates to lower secondary care costs. Comment on the literature relating to referral management.

1 How and why do referrals vary?

2 Are referrals avoidable?

3 How can referral rates be modified?

....

....

....

....

....

....

....

....

....

....

....

....

....

....

....

....

....

....

....

....

....

....

....

Question 5

How can burnout be avoided?

. . . .

. . . .

. . . .

. . . .

. . . .

. . . .

. . . .

. . . .

. . . .

. . . .

. . . .

. . . .

. . . .

. . . .

. . . .

. . . .

. . . .

. . . .

. . . .

. . . .

. . . .

. . . .

Question 6

Discuss the evidence relating to the following interventions in osteoarthritis:

1 Physiotherapy
2 Steroid injections
3 Dietary supplements
4 Topical and oral anti-inflammatories and analgesics

. . . .

. . . .

. . . .

. . . .

. . . .

. . . .

. . . .

. . . .

. . . .

. . . .

. . . .

. . . .

. . . .

. . . .

. . . .

. . . .

. . . .

. . . .

. . . .

. . . .

Question 7

As a result of an audit it has become clear that an excessive number of your patients fail to attend outpatient appointments after being referred by their GP. In a drive to improve access times you set up a working party to explore the causes of this. You wish the process to be evidence base]d.

1   Outline how you would gather the evidence

2   Read reference material 7.1a, part of a paper from the *British Journal of General Practice* entitled 'Patient, hospital and general practitioner characteristics associated with non-attendance: a cohort study' (with copyright permission from the *British Journal of General Practice* 2002; 52: 317–319). Comment on the strengths and weaknesses of the methodology of the study as presented

Reference material 7.1a

Method

The study used a prospective cohort approach. It was run in parallel with a randomised controlled trial of an intervention aimed to reduce non-attendance. Twenty-six GPs from 13 practices in Exeter, UK, enrolled all new referrals between January and May 1997 into the study.

The patients' age, sex, and referral specialty (surgery; obstetrics and gynaecology; medicine; orthopaedics; ophthalmology; ear, nose and throat or oral surgery; dermatology; psychiatry; or other) were extracted from the referral letter. The Jarman score, as a proxy measure of socioeconomic status, was calculated from the postcode. The interval between referral and appointment was calculated from the referral and reply letters. GP details were obtained from the Health Authority. Referral rates were calculated from the number of referrals made during the study and the list size calculated from practice details.

Attendance data were obtained from routine hospital datasets, cross-checked by examination of the GP records. Cancellations were considered as attendances for analysis. Attendance rates between specialties were compared using a χ^2 test. All variables (sex, age, Jarman score, interval to appointment, specialty, fundholding status, referral rate, possession of Membership of the Royal College of General Practitioners, and year of qualification of GP) were entered into a univariable analysis. Logistic regression was performed using non-attendance versus cancellation or attendance as the outcome measure. Those variables with a probability of the null hypothesis of less than 0.2 were entered into a multivariable analysis.

....
....
....
....
....
....
....
....
....
....
....
....
....
....
....
....
....
....
....
....
....
....
....
....
....
....
....
....
....
....
....
....

Question 8

1 Extracts from the results section of the paper referred to in the Question 7 are given in reference material 7.2a (with copyright permission from the *British Journal of General Practice*). What do you conclude from the results presented?

2 What other factors may explain the results seen?

Reference material 7.2a

Results

The study GPs enrolled 2078 patients; 1972 of these were sent appointments. No patient was lost to follow-up. Of those sent appointments, 106 patients (5.4%) failed to attend. Demographic details of the patients and information about their GP are shown in Table 1. The mean (standard deviation) referral rate during the study was 13.7 (6.3) per hundred patients per year. There were no significant differences in non-attendance between specialties. Men aged 16 to 35 years had a non-attendance rate of 21 %.

The univariable and multivariable results are shown in Table 2. Males, younger patients, those with a longer interval between referral and appointment, those with a higher Jarman score, and patients of a high-referring GP were all less likely to attend.

Reference material 7.2b

[See Tables 1 and 2 (overleaf)]

Table 1 Characteristics of non-attenders, compared with attenders and cancellations

Characteristic	Attenders and cancellations (n=1866)	Non-attenders (n=106)	Statistical test applied and significance
Percentage male (95% CI)	40.2 (38.0–42.5)	50.9 (41.0–60.8)	χ^2=4.9 P=0.03
Mean age in years (95% CI)	49.2 (48.1–50.2)	38.2 (34.2–42.1)	t-test=4.85 P<0.0001
Median (interquartile range) interval between referral and appointment (days)	50.7 (26.3–89.1)	110 (56.6–157.0)	Rank sum test P<0.0001
Percentage from a fundholding general practitioner (95% CI)	23.9 (22.0–25.9)	29.2 (20.8–38.9)	χ^2=1.6 P=0.21
Percentage from a general practitioner with MRCGP[a] (95% CI)	73.9 (71.7–75.8)	79.3 (70.3–86.5)	χ^2=1.5 P=0.22

[a] Membership of the Royal College of General Practitioners

Table 2 Multivariable analysis of characteristics of non-attendance

Characteristic	Univariable analysis		Multivariable analaysis	
	Odds ratio (CI)	Significance	Odds ratio (CI)	Significance
Male sex	1.60 (1.08–2.38)	0.02	1.65 (1.09–2.50)	0.02
Age	0.98[a] (0.97–0.99)	<0.001	0.98[a] (0.97–0.99)	<0.001
Jarman score	1.02 (1.01–1.03)	0.003	1.02 (1.01–1.03)	0.008
Interval to appointment	1.06[b] (1.05–1.08)	<0.001	1.07[b] (1.05–1.09)	<0.001
Referral rate of GP	1.03[c] (1.00–1.05)	0.06	1.03[c] (1.00–1.06)	0.05

[a] For a one-year increase in age. [b] For a one-week increase in interval. [c] For an increase of one referral per hundred patients per year.

Question 9

1   How does the literature contribute to the diagnosis and initial assessment of chronic obstructive pulmonary disease (COPD)?

2   Describe the step-wise use of initial therapy for COPD with an algorithm

3   How does the literature contribute to the management of exacerbations of COPD?

. . . .

. . . .

. . . .

. . . .

. . . .

. . . .

. . . .

. . . .

. . . .

. . . .

. . . .

. . . .

. . . .

. . . .

. . . .

. . . .

. . . .

. . . .

. . . .

Question 10

While looking at ways to improve the care of patients with epilepsy in your practice, you come across the paper 'A pragmatic randomised controlled trial of a prompt and reminder card in the care of people with epilepsy' (with permission from the *British Journal of General Practice* 2002; 52: 93–98; reference material 7.3a).

1 Comment on the strengths and weaknesses of the method described

2 Comment on the results of the trial (shown in Tables 1, 2 and 3 of reference material 7.3b)

3 Comment on possible reasons for these results

Reference material 7.3a

Method

Protocol

Practices in four areas of Greater Manchester (Stockport, South Manchester, Salford and Trafford, and Bury and Rochdale) were randomly selected and approached to participate in this study. The study was conducted between April 1997 and August 1999. Adults with 'active' epilepsy (either a seizure recorded in the medical records in the past two years or being on anticonvulsant medication for epilepsy) on the list of consenting GPs were eligible to participate. Temporary residents, individuals with severe learning disability, and children (individuals under 16 years of age) were excluded.

Intervention

The intervention consisted of an evidence-based epilepsy prompt and reminder card for GPs to complete. The card had two main parts: first, 'prompts' to collect key clinical information about an individual's epilepsy; and secondly, evidence-based information ('reminders') on which to then base any subsequent patient management decision. The final version of the prompt and reminder card was passport-sized, bright yellow in colour, and consisted of nine sections (including seizure frequency and pattern, seizure classification, medication, side-effects and indications for medication withdrawal, checking serum levels, information provision, and monitoring).

Assignment

The study was a pragmatic randomised trial. Practices were stratified into small (fewer than three partners in practice) or large (three or more partners in the practice). Using a random number table, practices were either allocated to the 'control' group, to the 'doctor-held card' group (where the card was inserted into the patients' records) or to the 'patient-held card' group (where the patient held the card). The card was used opportunistically over the course of one year for most subjects.

The primary outcome measures were recording of seizure frequency and self-reported seizure frequency in the previous year. Secondary outcome measures were the retrieval rate and completion rate of the epilepsy card, the proportion of patients on monotherapy with anticonvulsants, the proportion of patients reporting medication side-effects, whether serum levels of anticonvulsants were checked appropriately, the levels of patient satisfaction with GP care, and level of satisfaction with information provision by the GP.

The outcome measures used were items from the Liverpool Assessment Battery and information recorded in GP medical records. The Liverpool Assessment Battery comprises several scales (including the Seizure Severity scale, the HAD questionnaire) and individual items to measure the quality of life and the quality of care for people with epilepsy. Baseline questionnaire data were collected before randomisation with further questionnaire data being collected after the intervention. Data from medical records were extracted on two separate occasions (for baseline year and intervention year information).

Ethical approval was obtained from the relevant ethical committees (South Manchester, Bury and Rochdale, Salford and Trafford, and Stockport) prior to commencing recruitment.

Statistical methods

The sample size calculations were based on an estimated 10% reduction in seizure frequency and recorded seizure frequency (with 80% power and a 5% significance level). As randomisation was by practice, an intra-class correlation coefficient of 0.02 was estimated for outcome measures to account for clustering within practices. Previous studies had found that each GP had about 10 patients with epilepsy and that the average practice size was 3.5 GPs. It was calculated that 20 practices in the three arms of the study with 600 patients in each arm would yield enough power to detect this difference in seizure frequency.

Statistical analyses were based on generalised estimating equations, in which the intra-cluster correlation is accounted for using an exchangeable correlation model assuming a logistic model for binary outcomes. Prior to analysis, covariates that were potential predictors of outcome were identified and included in the model to improve efficiency and reduce chance bias. Analyses were carried out using the STATA statistical software. Where baseline covariates were missing, an additional 'missing' category level was used or an imputed value was assigned for continuous variables.

For each outcome, comparison was made between the three groups by means of a 0.05 two-tailed significance level using a Wald χ^2 test. Where there was evidence of difference between groups, pair-wise tests were carried out between the control and each of the intervention groups using a 0.025 two-tailed significance level. Analysis was done on an intention-to-treat basis.

Reference material 7.3b

[Tables 1–2 (overleaf)]

Table 1 Recording of seizure frequency, either in medical records or on card in previous year

	Control	Doctor held	Patient held	Overall
Baseline				
In medical notes % (n)	37.8 (143/378)	36.6 (186/508)	36.5 (133/364)	37 (462/1250)
Intervention year				
Medical notes or card % (n)	42.8 (157/367)	57.4 (281/489)	44.6 (158/356)	49.3 (596/1210)
Adjusted[a] odds ratio relative to control group (95% CI)	—	1.82 (1.23–2.69)	1.16 (0.76–1.77)	—
Wald χ^2 comparing intervention with control[a] (one degree of freedom)	—	$P=0.003$	$P=0.49$	$P=0.0058$[b]

Intra-class correlation coefficient = 0.051.
[a] Adjusted for baseline recording of seizure, health problems, and visit to specialist in baseline year.
[b] Wald χ^2 comparing three arms (two degrees of freedom).

Table 2 Reported seizure frequency during the baseline and intervention year

	Control	Doctor held	Patient held	Overall
Seizure status in previous year				
Baseline year				
Seizure free % (n)	48.3 (181/374)	51.6 (247/479)	52.0 (179/344)	50.7 (607/1197)
Intervention year				
Seizure free % (n)	51.5 (151/293)	56.0 (219/391)	58.1 (158/272)	55.2 (528/956)
Adjusted[a] odds ratio relative to control group (95% CI)	—	1.33 (0.83–2.13)	1.47 (0.88–2.46)	—
Wald χ^2 comparing intervention with control[a] (one degree of freedom)	—	$P=0.238$	$P=0.137$	$P=0.297$[b]

Intra-class correlation coefficient = 0.022.
[a] Adjusted for baseline seizure frequency, health problems, age, and visit to specialist in baseline year.
[b] Wald χ^2 comparing three arms (two degrees of freedom).

Table 3 Summary of other results on medication use, side-effects, and monitoring and on satisfaction with GP care during the baseline and intervention year

	Control	Doctor held	Patient held
Medication use			
On more than one epilepsy drug in baseline year % (n)	28.8 (106/368)	28.1 (131/467)	32.1 (110/343)
On more than one epilepsy drug in intervention year % (n)	28.9 (83/287)	30.3 (113/373)	29.9 (79/264)
Adjusted[a] odds ratio relative to control group (95% CI)	–	0.76 (0.41–1.44)	1.51 (0.74–3.07)
Wald χ^2 comparing intervention with control[a] (one degree of freedom)		$P = 0.401$	$P = 0.253$
Medication side effects			
Medication side effects reported by patient during baseline year % (n)	52.8 (182/345)	50.8 (229/450)	53.2 (173/326)
Medication side effects reported by patient during intervention year % (n)	43.6 (120/275)	49.3 (182/369)	50.8 (125/246)
Adjusted[b] odds ratio relative to control group (95% CI)	–	1.54 (1.10–2.17)	1.60 (1.10–2.32)
Wald χ^2 comparing intervention with control[b] (one degree of freedom)		$P = 0.013$	$P = 0.016$
Checking of phenytoin serum levels in previous year (for those patients on phenytoin)			
Phenytoin serum levels checked in baseline year % (n)	31.2 (39/125)	28.1 (52/185)	32.6 (42/129)
Phenytoin serum levels checked in intervention year % (n)	31.5 (34/108)	28.7 (45/157)	39.2 (40/102)
Adjusted[c] odds ratio relative to control group (95% CI)	–	0.93 (0.44–1.97)	1.37 (0.61–3.09)
Wald χ^2 comparing intervention with control[c] (one degree of freedom)		$P = 0.851$	$P = 0.447$
Satisfaction with information provision by the GP in previous year (for those patients who reported seeing the GP in the previous year)			
Satisfied with information provided by the GP in baseline year % (n)	67.7 (195/288)	64.4 (239/371)	65.1 (183/281)
Satisfied with information provided by the GP in intervention year % (n)	76.1 (175/230)	66.0 (195/295)	76.2 (162/213)
Adjusted[d] odds ratio relative to control group (95% CI)	–	0.57 (0.38–0.86)	0.98 (0.62–1.54)
Wald χ^2 comparing intervention with control[d] (one degree of freedom)		$P = 0.006$	$P = 0.943$

Table 3 (continued)

	Control	Doctor held	Patient held
Rated GP care of their epilepsy as high (either excellent or good) (for those patients who reported seeing the GP in the previous year)			
Rated GP care of their epilepsy as high in baseline year % (n)	77.2 (223/289)	76.7 (284/370)	77.5 (217/280)
Rated GP care of their epilepsy as high in intervention year % (n)	79.0 (181/229)	73.6 (220/299)	83.6 (179/214)
Adjusted[e] odds ratio relative to control group (95% CI)	–	0.70 (0.45–1.07)	1.35 (0.80–2.21)
Wald χ^2 comparing intervention with control[e] (one degree of freedom)	–	$P = 0.10$	$P = 0.27$

[a] Adjusted for baseline number of epilepsy drugs. Tonic clonic seizures. GP attendance's intervention year. [b] Adjusted for baseline presence of medication side-effects. Other long-term illness. Age. [c] Adjusted for baseline checking of phenytoin levels and age. [d] Adjusted for baseline information provision and age. [e] Adjusted for baseline satisfaction with care and age.

....
....
....
....
....
....
....
....
....
....
....
....
....
....
....
....
....
....
....
....
....
....
....
....
....
....
....

Question 11

Discuss the impact of deprivation on general practice.

. . . .
. . . .
. . . .
. . . .
. . . .
. . . .
. . . .
. . . .
. . . .
. . . .
. . . .
. . . .
. . . .
. . . .
. . . .
. . . .
. . . .
. . . .
. . . .
. . . .
. . . .
. . . .
. . . .
. . . .
. . . .

Question 12

A 21-year-old girl and her boyfriend come to you for the morning-after pill. They both have Down's syndrome and attend a local daycare centre. What issues does this raise, and how would you proceed?

. . . .

. . . .

. . . .

. . . .

. . . .

. . . .

. . . .

. . . .

. . . .

. . . .

. . . .

. . . .

. . . .

. . . .

. . . .

. . . .

. . . .

. . . .

. . . .

. . . .

. . . .

. . . .

Paper 8

Question 1

Hannah, a normally fit and active 3-year-old, is brought to you by her parents. She is lethargic, dehydrated and smells ketotic. A fingerprick BM shows a blood glucose of 22. What are your aims now and in the future?

. . . .

. . . .

. . . .

. . . .

. . . .

. . . .

. . . .

. . . .

. . . .

. . . .

. . . .

. . . .

. . . .

. . . .

. . . .

. . . .

. . . .

Question 2

'Growing old gracefully' – how can general practice meet the needs of elderly people?

. . . .

. . . .

. . . .

. . . .

. . . .

. . . .

. . . .

. . . .

. . . .

. . . .

. . . .

. . . .

. . . .

. . . .

. . . .

. . . .

. . . .

. . . .

. . . .

. . . .

. . . .

. . . .

. . . .

Question 3

The NSF for Elderly People and Stroke places new emphasis on the prevention and treatment of stroke. See reference material 8.1a, an extract from the paper 'Use of ramipril in preventing stroke: double blind randomised trial' (with copyright permission from *British Medical Journal* 2002; 324: 699).

1   Comment on the methodology of the trial

2   Comment on the results in Table 1 of reference material 8.1b

3   Comment on the statement from the conclusion 'Widespread use of an angiotensin converting enzyme inhibitor such as ramipril in patients at high risk of stroke is likely to have a major impact on public health' ('The Heart Outcomes Prevention Evaluation Study Investigation', *N Eng J Med* 2000; 342: 145–153, Jan 20, 2000)

Reference material 8.1a

Design and methods

The HOPE study was a double blind randomised trial with a two by two factorial design, in which participants were randomised to receive up to 10 mg of ramipril, 400 IU of vitamin E, both, or matching placebos. We provide a brief outline here.

Participants

Participants were aged 55 or over and were at high risk of cardiovascular events because of previous coronary artery disease, cerebrovascular disease, or peripheral arterial disease or diabetes plus one additional risk factor. Patients were excluded if they were taking either an angiotensin converting enzyme inhibitor or vitamin E; had heart failure or a known left ventricular ejection fraction of less than 0.40, known proteinuria, or uncontrolled hypertension; or had had a previous stroke or a myocardial infarction less than one month before enrolment in the study. Informed consent was obtained from all participants before enrolment in the study, and the study was approved by the ethics committee at each centre.

Intervention

Eligible patients entered a run-in phase in which they received 2.5 mg ramipril daily for 7–10 days, after which serum creatinine and potassium levels were measured. Participants then started a 10–14 day course of placebo. Those who tolerated and adhered to this regimen were then randomised to receive either placebo or 2.5 mg ramipril daily for one week, followed by placebo or 5.0 mg ramipril for a further three weeks. One month after randomisation the patient's serum creatinine and potassium were measured; if these were satisfactory the patient continued on either placebo or 10 mg ramipril for the remainder of the study. Participants were seen after six months and then every six months until the end of the study, with an average follow up of 4.5 years.

Of the 10 576 patients who entered the run-in phase, 1035 were not randomised because of non-adherence, side effects, or withdrawal of consent; 244 patients were entered into a substudy of 2.5 mg ramipril and are not included in this paper. Outcome results were available on 9539 (99.9%) of the 9541 patients randomised. The first participant was recruited in December 1993. The originally scheduled completion date was November 1999, but the ramipril arm of the study was terminated early (April 1999) because of clear benefit.

Outcome measures

The primary outcome was the composite end point of myocardial infarction, stroke, or cardiovascular death. The individual components of this composite end point were analysed separately. All outcomes were adjudicated by a central committee. This analysis focuses on stroke. Investigators reported the occurrences of stroke or transient ischaemic attack at follow up visits. For every stroke reported, information on the stroke, including symptoms and functional impairment, was documented.

The investigators used a simple six point scale to record if there was full recovery, persistent symptoms, some functional impairment, functional impairment necessitating the assistance of others to perform activities of daily living, or inability to perform activities of daily living even with help at seven days or at discharge if earlier. Discharge summaries, consultation notes, and results of computed tomography or magnetic resonance imaging were documented. A central committee adjudicated all strokes on the basis of predetermined definitions. Classification of a stroke as either ischaemic or haemorrhagic was confirmed by computed tomography or magnetic resonance imaging within 14 days of onset or by autopsy. All other strokes were classified as being of uncertain aetiology. Computed tomography, magnetic resonance imaging, or autopsy results were obtained for 84% of strokes.

Blood pressure was measured at entry to the study, after two years, and at the end of the study. Two measurements were taken on each arm after the patient had been supine for five minutes. The lowest measurements on each arm were averaged to obtain the systolic and diastolic values that were recorded.

Statistical analysis

The study had 90% power to detect a 13.5% reduction in relative risk for the primary outcome, with an annual event rate of 4% in 9000 patients studied for five years. Assuming a stroke rate of 1.2% per year in the control group for five years, the study had 80% power to detect a 22.0% reduction in the relative risk of stroke with a two sided α level of 0.05 in an intention to treat analysis. We estimated survival curves according to the Kaplan-Meier procedure and compared treatments by using the log rank test. Because of the factorial design, we stratified all analyses for the randomisation to vitamin E or placebo. We conducted subgroup analyses by using tests for interactions in the Cox regression model. We used this model to estimate the reduction in relative risk and the 95% confidence intervals associated with ramipril treatment in unadjusted analyses and after controlling for changes in blood pressure.

The data and safety monitoring board monitored the study. Monitoring boundaries for the study were four standard deviations between the two groups in terms of benefit of ramipril in the first half of the study and three standard deviations in the second half. For harm, the boundaries were three standard deviations in the first half of the study and two standard deviations in the second half. Because of clear benefit, the study was terminated on 22 March 1999.

Study organisation

The study was conducted in 267 hospital clinics in 19 countries. It was coordinated by the Canadian Cardiovascular Collaboration in Hamilton, Canada.

Reference material 8.1b

Table 1 Impact of ramipril on stroke subdivided by non-fatal and fatal stroke, subtype of stroke, and presence or absence of functional impairment. Values are numbers (percentages) unless stated otherwise

Outcome	Ramipril (n=4645)	Placebo (n=4652)	Relative risk (95% CI)
Total strokes	156 (3.4)	226 (4.9)	0.68 (0.56 to 0.84)
Non-fatal:	139 (3.0)	182 (3.9)	0.76 (0.61 to 0.94)
No functional impairment	49 (1.1)	80 (1.7)	0.61 (0.43 to 0.87)
Some functional impairment*	85 (1.8)	108 (2.3)	0.78 (0.59 to 1.04)
Fatal	17 (0.4)	44 (1.0)	0.39 (0.22 to 0.67)
Subtype of stroke			
Ischaemic	101 (2.2)	157 (3.4)	0.64 (0.50 to 0.82)
Non-ischaemic†:	63 (1.4)	78 (1.7)	0.80 (0.57 to 1.12)
Haemorrhagic	12 (0.26)	16 (0.34)	0.74 (0.35 to 1.57)
Uncertain aetiology	52 (1.1)	65 (1.4)	0.79 (0.55 to 1.14)

* Any impairment from functional impairment that does not limit daily activities to assistance needed for all activities of daily living.
† Stroke of haemorrhagic or uncertain aetiology.

. . . .

. . . .

. . . .

. . . .

. . . .

. . . .

. . . .

. . . .

. . . .

. . . .

. . . .

. . . .

. . . .

. . . .

. . . .

. . . .

. . . .

. . . .

. . . .

. . . .

. . . .

. . . .

. . . .

. . . .

. . . .

. . . .

. . . .

. . . .

. . . .

. . . .

. . . .

. . . .

. . . .

Question 4

The practice receptionist points out that there seem to be a large number of patients not attending appointments. What do you need to consider when looking at this problem?

. . . .

. . . .

. . . .

. . . .

. . . .

. . . .

. . . .

. . . .

. . . .

. . . .

. . . .

. . . .

. . . .

. . . .

. . . .

. . . .

. . . .

. . . .

. . . .

. . . .

. . . .

. . . .

Question 5

A 30-year-old woman with a BMI of 32 comes to see you requesting a prescription for slimming drugs which she read about in a magazine. What issues does this consultation raise?

Question 6

Discuss the available evidence regarding screening and prevention of type 2 diabetes.

. . . .

. . . .

. . . .

. . . .

. . . .

. . . .

. . . .

. . . .

. . . .

. . . .

. . . .

. . . .

. . . .

. . . .

. . . .

. . . .

. . . .

. . . .

. . . .

. . . .

. . . .

. . . .

. . . .

Question 7

Comment on the evidence relating to the management of hay fever.

....

....

....

....

....

....

....

....

....

....

....

....

....

....

....

....

....

....

....

....

....

....

....

....

Question 8

Discuss how doctors can identify their learning needs.

. . . .

. . . .

. . . .

. . . .

. . . .

. . . .

. . . .

. . . .

. . . .

. . . .

. . . .

. . . .

. . . .

. . . .

. . . .

. . . .

. . . .

. . . .

. . . .

. . . .

. . . .

. . . .

. . . .

Question 9

One of your practice nurses wishes to go on a course on screening for prostate cancer. What issues does this raise and how would you address her request?

. . . .
. . . .
. . . .
. . . .
. . . .
. . . .
. . . .
. . . .
. . . .
. . . .
. . . .
. . . .
. . . .
. . . .
. . . .
. . . .
. . . .
. . . .
. . . .
. . . .
. . . .
. . . .
. . . .
. . . .

Question 10

**Discuss the diagnosis and management of eating disorders.
Give evidence to support your views.**

....

....

....

....

....

....

....

....

....

....

....

....

....

....

....

....

....

....

....

....

....

....

....

....

....

....

Question 11

  1 **What are the problems encountered in studying therapies in arthritis?**

     See reference material 8.2a, an extract from the paper 'Long-term effects of glucosamine sulphate on osteoarthritis progression: a randomised, placebo-controlled clinical trial'. Reprinted with permission from Elsevier Science (*Lancet* 2001; 357: 251–256) and answer the following questions:

  2 **Comment on the methodology described in reference material 8.2a**

  3 **Comment on the results in Tables 2 and 3 of reference material 8.2b**

Reference material 8.2a

Methods

Study design and selection of patients

We recruited patients from the outpatient clinic of the Bone and Cartilage Metabolism Research Unit of the University Hospital Centre in Liege, Belgium. Inclusion criteria were age over 50 years and primary knee osteoarthritis of the medial femorotibial compartment, diagnosed according to the clinical and radiological criteria of the American College of Rheumatology. Disease severity was graded on the basis of the Kellgren and Lawrence radiographic system. Major exclusion criteria were: history or active presence of other rheumatic diseases that could be responsible for secondary osteoarthritis; severe articular inflammation as confirmed by physical examination (excluded also by erythrocyte sedimentation rate < 40 mm/h and serum rheumatoid factor titre $<1{:}40$); traumatic knee lesions; overweight defined as a body mass index >30; substantial abnormalities in haematological, hepatic, renal, or metabolic functions; and intra-articular or systemic corticosteroids in the 3 months preceding enrolment. The study was approved by the ethics committee of the University of Liege and all patients gave their oral and written informed consent to participate.

Treatment assignment

Crystalline glucosamine sulphate (Dona, Viartril-S, or Xicil, Rotta Research Group, Monza, Italy) is a defined pure substance that is synthesised from chitin, and in which glucosamine sulphate, chloride, and sodium ions are present in stoichiometric ratios of 2:1:2:2. The net content of glucosamine sulphate in the dose form (powder for oral solution, with standard inactive excipients) is 1500 mg. This product has been approved at this once daily dosage as a prescription treatment for osteoarthritis in many countries in Europe and elsewhere.

Patients were randomly assigned to receive 1500 mg of glucosamine sulphate or placebo once daily for 3 years. For rescue analgesia, patients were allowed access to paracetamol in 500 mg tablets, or to one of the following NSAIDs (the most used in Belgium at the time of the trial): diclofenac in 50 mg tablets, piroxicam in 20 mg capsules, or proglumetacin in 150 mg tablets. Use of the rescue medications was recorded by the patients in a diary, with appropriate washout – ie, at least five half-lives of the selected medication were allowed before symptom assessment. Compliance with study treatment was established by asking the patients about missed doses and by counting unused sachets. No other co-interventions for osteoarthritis were allowed.

The randomisation list was generated by computer in blocks of four, and patients received their randomisation number in chronological order. The principal investigator was provided with individual envelopes, each containing patient codes, thus concealing treatment assignment.

Outcome measures

The primary outcome measure for joint structural changes was represented by the mean joint-space width of the medial compartment of the tibiofemoral joint. Weightbearing, anteroposterior, separate radiographs of each knee were taken at baseline, 1, and 3 years by a standardised technique. In brief, patients stood with their knees fully extended and the posterior aspect of the knee in contact with the vertical cassette. The lower limbs were rotated until the patella was centralised over the lower end of the femur. Feet were positioned a small distance apart: foot maps were used for repositioning the patient. The X-ray beam was centred on the joint space and parallel to the tibial plateau. Fluoroscopy was used to correct lower limb positioning and X-ray beam alignment. The focus to film distance was 110 cm.

We digitised the radiographs and did the image analysis automatically by a validated system, which located the proximal and distal joint margins excluding outlier points and calculated the mean joint-space width of the medial and lateral compartments of the tibiofemoral joint. We calculated the mean (SD) short-term and long-term coefficient of variation of this system for reproducing measurements as 1.82% (1.29) and 1.62% (1.31), respectively, for the medial compartment, which is in good agreement with the 1.84% coefficient of variation reported in the original validation of this method. All radiographs obtained in a single radiological unit in Liege were measured in London by a single reader unaware of treatment assignment. A further masked analysis was visual determination of the minimum joint-space width – ie, at the narrowest point – with a 0.1 mm graduated magnifying lens.

We assessed symptoms of osteoarthritis by the Western Ontario and McMaster Universities (WOMAC) osteoarthritis index, a validated, disease-specific questionnaire addressing severity of joint pain (five questions), stiffness (two questions), and limitation of physical function (17 questions), and referring to the 48h before assessment. The visual analogue scale version of the index was used – ie, with the patient assessing each question by a 100 mm visual analogue scale, and the total index score being represented by the sum of the 24 component item scores. A higher WOMAC score represents worse symptom severity, with 2400 mm being the worst possible total score.

Secondary outcome measures were use of rescue medications as recorded in a daily diary; withdrawal rates; occurrence of adverse events; and routine safety laboratory tests, including testing for glucose homoeostasis assessed by fasting glucose concentrations at yearly intervals in all patients still receiving the study treatment.

Statistical analysis

We calculated sample size on the basis of the recommendations available at the time of study planning, of a 0.5 mm target difference in joint-space narrowing between groups after 3 years, given the validation data of the digital image analysis technique adopted as the principal outcome. We calculated that a sample size of at least 60 patients in each group would give a power of 80% in detecting such a difference at the 5% significance level. We increased the sample size to at least 100 patients per group to allow an up to 40% dropout rate.

The primary efficacy outcome measure for structure modification was joint-space narrowing in the signal joint – ie, the change in joint-space width after 3 years in the narrowest medial tibiofemoral joint compartment at enrolment. The medial tibiofemoral joint space is preferred in clinical trials, as opposed to the lateral space, since this is the area that is subjected to the greatest pressure and thus the most osteoarthritis cartilage loss, and for which outcome measures are better validated. The 3-year % change in the total WOMAC score was taken for the primary assessment of symptom modification, with the final changes in the pain, physical function, and stiffness subscales analysed as secondary endpoints.

Results were expressed as difference between the final group means and 95% CI, with p values based on analysis of variance. All primary efficacy analyses were done on patients who completed the 3-year observation period, and by intention-to-treat analysis for all randomised patients. Every

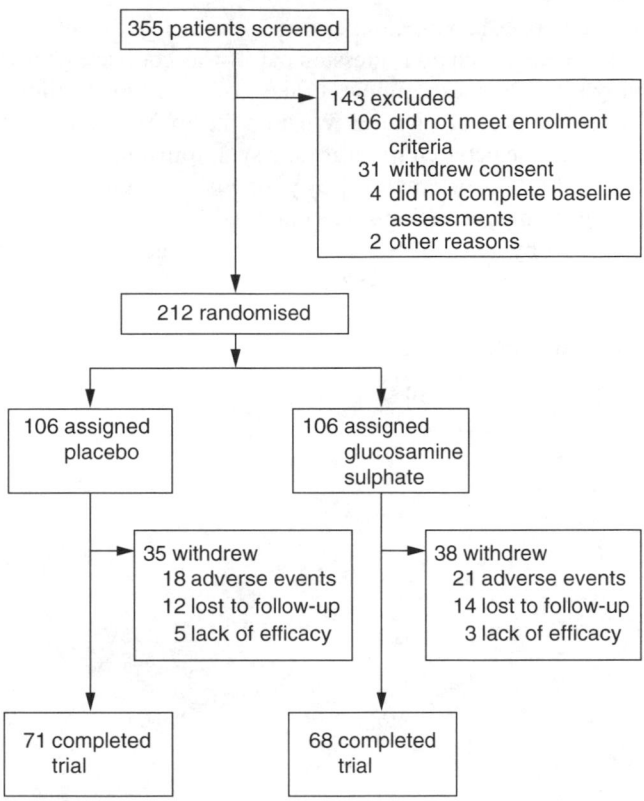

355 patients screened

143 excluded
    106 did not meet enrolment
        criteria
    31 withdrew consent
    4 did not complete baseline
        assessments
    2 other reasons

212 randomised

106 assigned
placebo

106 assigned
glucosamine
sulphate

35 withdrew
    18 adverse events
    12 lost to follow-up
    5 lack of efficacy

38 withdrew
    21 adverse events
    14 lost to follow-up
    3 lack of efficacy

71 completed
trial

68 completed
trial

Figure 1   Trial profile

effort was made to carry out the final examinations after 3 years, regardless of patient's compliance or whether the patient was still on the study treatment. When this was not possible, the intention-to-treat analysis was carried out according to three different approaches. First, we did a worst scenario analysis in which a poor outcome was assigned to patients in whom the final 3-year assessment was not completed, corresponding to the average change recorded in patients in the placebo group who were assessed for 3 years. For consistency we also used the last observation carried forward approach, and to avoid repeatedly assigning the same value to a series of missing values we used the random sampling method. In the random sampling approach, missing endpoint values were replaced with values selected randomly from the distribution of all known endpoint values – ie, glucosamine sulphate and placebo combined. To lower sampling error, 50 such datasets were constructed, analysed independently by analysis of variance and the median of the significance values was taken.

Among secondary analyses, we arbitrarily defined a cutoff point for marked structural damage progression as a joint-space narrowing of more than 0.5 mm, based on previous reports – the proportion of all randomised patients reaching such a progression cutoff was compared between groups by the χ^2 test. The mean number of days of rescue medication intake was assessed by analysis of variance. We used the Spearman correlation test to assess correlation between structure and symptom outcomes. Adverse event and dropout rates were analysed by χ^2 or Fisher's exact tests, as appropriate. Baseline characteristics were compared by the χ^2 test for categorical variables and by analysis of variance for continuous data. All reported p values are two sided with $\alpha = 0.05$.

Reference material 8.2b

[Tables 2 and 3 (opposite)]

Table 2 Average (95% CI) joint-space narrowing after 3 years

	Patients assessed for 3 years				Intention-to-treat analysis			
	Placebo (n=71)	Glucosamine sulphate (n=68)	Difference (95% CI)	p	Placebo (n=106)	Glucosamine sulphate (n=106)	Difference (95% CI)	p
Mean joint-space narrowing (mm)	-0.31 (-0.57 to -0.04)	0.07 (-0.17 to 0.32)	0.38 (0.02 to 0.73)	0.038	-0.31 (-0.48 to -0.13)	-0.06 (-0.22 to 0.09)	0.24 (0.01 to 0.48)	0.043
Minimum joint-space narrowing (mm)	-0.40 (-0.64 to -0.17)	0.11 (-0.10 to 0.33)	0.51 (0.20 to 0.83)	0.002	-0.40 (-0.56 to -0.24)	-0.07 (-0.22 to 0.07)	0.33 (0.12 to 0.54)	0.003

Table 3 Average (95% CI) total WOMAC percent change after 3 years

	Patients assessed for 3 years				Intention-to-treat analysis			
	Placebo (n=71)	Glucosamine sulphate (n=68)	Difference (95% CI)	p	Placebo (n=106)	Glucosamine sulphate (n=106)	Difference (95% CI)	p
Total WOMAC % change	9.8% (-14.6 to 34.3%)	-24.3% (-37.0 to -11.6%)	34.1% (6.4 to 61.8%)	0.016	9.8% (-6.2 to 25.8%)	-11.7% (-20.3 to -3.2%)	21.6% (3.5 to 39.6%)	0.020

Question 12

See reference material 8.3a, an extract from the paper 'The effect of GP telephone triage on numbers seeking same day appointments' (with copyright permission from *British Journal of General Practice* 2002; 52: 390–392). In terms of relevance to managing demand in UK general practice, discuss the methodology and results of this study.

Reference material 8.3a

Method

The study took place from July 1999 to June 2000 and was carried out in a group practice located in a market town, with a list size of 7200, and four GPs. Levels of deprivation were close to the national average (Jarman score = −4.26). The practice introduced a telephone consultation policy whereby all patients requesting same-day appointments were told that a GP would telephone them later. GPs were asked to log the outcome of these telephone consultations. A patient satisfaction survey was sent to all patients who had received such a telephone call over a one-month period during the intervention. Numbers attending out-of-hours were compared with previous years.

Statistical analysis

Numbers attending the surgery for routine and 'extra' appointments over two years (1997 and 1998) were entered onto an SPSS database. Regression analysis was performed to determine if there was a pattern to the demand for 'extra' appointments and if this pattern had a temporal basis. These data were used to assess the impact of a telephone triage intervention. To determine the impact of the telephone triage intervention, linear regression was performed on the logged counts with a harmonic term to allow for seasonality and a dummy variable which takes the value zero for pre-intervention and one for post-intervention. The analysis was performed using autoregression in SPSS to allow for serial correlation and linear regression using the Durbin-Watson statistic, to test whether serial correlation had been successfully removed.

Results

A plot of the 'extra' appointments for 1997 and 1998 suggested a seasonal pattern. A regression of the number of extra appointments required against time was reasonably well fitted (adjusted $R^2 = 0.40$). A reduction of 39.3% in the demand for face-to-face appointments was observed during the intervention phase as shown in Figure 1.

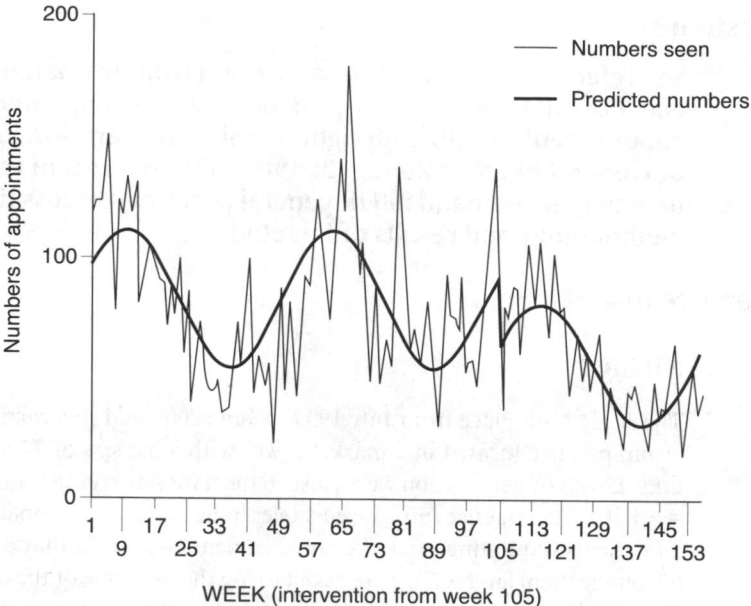

Figure 1   Effect of telephone consultations on demand for 'extras'

Patient satisfaction survey

A 74% response rate to the postal questionnaire was recorded (111 responses in total). The majority of patients were satisfied or very satisfied with the outcome of the telephone consultation (98%) and most (84%) said they would be happy to receive this service in similar circumstances in the future (95% CI = 76 to 90). Patient use of out-of-hours services showed a drop in the study period.

Use of telephone

The total number of calls in the second half of the study period from January 2000 to June 2000 was 3680, with an average duration of less than two minutes. Ninety-three per cent had a duration of less than five minutes. The telephone bills increased by £200 per quarter over the study period. The total number of telephone calls recorded during one month in the second half of the study period was 615. The outcomes as recorded by the GPs in their telephone consultation diaries over this month are shown in Table 1 (outcomes not mutually exclusive, ie some telephone consultations resulted in more than one outcome).

Table 1 Outcome of telephone consultations

Outcome	Numbers (percentage of total)
Same-day appointment offered	266 (43.3)
Advice only	180 (29.3)
Prescription offered without face-to-face consultation	138 (22.4)
Visit	15 (2.4)
Routine appointment offered (not same day)	25 (4.1)
Appointment with nurse	8 (0.8)
Patient not available to speak to doctor	7 (1.1)

Discussion

Our study suggests that it is possible to use telephone consultations as an alternative to face-to-face consultations for patients seeking same-day appointments. More than one in five patients were offered a prescription without a clinical examination. All patients receiving a prescription who responded to the questionnaire expressed satisfaction with the outcome of their telephone consultation.

The role of nurse practitioners for patients seeking same-day appointments or in telephone triage has been endorsed recently. However, the management of patients seeking same-day appointments in our study was streamlined by GPs without diverting nursing staff away from other roles. It has been argued that the increasing promotion of nurse practitioners to deal with patients who need a same-day appointment might promote inequality rather than improve primary care. This paper suggests an alternative for those who might wish to retain access to GPs on a same-day basis. However, there is a financial cost to offering this service, as the practice would have to pay more in telephone charges.

....
....
....
....
....
....
....
....
....
....
....
....
....
....
....
....
....
....
....
....
....
....
....
....
....
....
....
....

Part 3:
Answers

Paper 1

Answer 1

The new GMS contract has promised a revolution in out-of-hours care. Discuss the implications of this change for all the stakeholders.

Implications for doctors

Personal

- Opportunity for some to stop doing out of hours, allowing time to pursue other interests, devote time to family and recharge batteries.
- Opportunity for others to increase earnings and fund lifestyle. Need to acknowledge limitations and need for time off when planning work.

Professional

- Loss of status as the caring family doctor to whom your patients turn to when in need. Will no longer have 24-hour responsibility which may cause resentment.
- Some doctors may lose skills used in out-of-hours care, such as telephone triage and minor injury work. Other doctors may have an opportunity to develop these skills and even work as full-time out-of-hours doctors. Doctors who feel ill at ease seeing unfamiliar patients in unfamiliar surroundings will find it a relief.
- Those doctors who continue to do out of hours care may find they need to embrace new ways of working with wider members of the health service, eg district nurses, paramedics and NHS Direct. A reflective approach to learning is essential to meet the educational challenge. This part of work will need to be considered as part of appraisal and revalidation.

Work patterns/administration

- Need to publicise out-of-hours contact points.
- Monday morning and Friday afternoon likely to be busier as patients try to see doctors within the working week.

- Need to consider within partnership agreement implications of GPs 'moonlighting' out of hours. What is acceptable?

Financial

- Cost of opting out £6000–£9000 per year. Earnings from sessions are superannuable. Loss of casualty payments when opting-out for those GPs covering minor injury units.
- Potential differential defence organisation subscriptions in future.
- In a buyers' market GPs are able to charge what they want to in some areas.

Implications for patients

- Will not be able to access local doctor easily. Might have to accept that if they wish to see a doctor they may have to travel to a treatment centre.
- May find they have to accept seeing a paramedic or district nurse first. They may find this difficult if they are used to seeing a doctor at a time of their choosing.
- Making multiple telephone calls to access healthcare may be a deterrent. NHS Direct may be used as a triage – which is not known for prompt callbacks. May limit access to healthcare – at present can ring NHS Direct or GP service for second opinion.
- According to the Carson report recommendations, patients will receive full treatment courses at the time of contact, saving trips to chemist to collect prescriptions.
- Patients with transport problems may not be able to attend treatment centres and may not receive equality of care.
- More likely to receive telephone advice or have non-urgent problems deferred.

Implications for PCT

- Cost of running service likely to be far in excess of money recouped from GPs. In the absence of extra funding from the DOH this may affect other services.
- Need to plan ahead and implement change early. Training needs for nurses and paramedics, IT needs.
- Risk management burden passes to PCT instead of doctors.

Implications for the Department of Health

- Costing at £6000–£9000 per GP set to make opt-out realistic, but PCTs not funded sufficiently so will inevitably divert funds or beg for more.

- Diversion of experienced nurses to out-of-hours care from other areas will affect other services, eg A&E.
- Diversion of experienced paramedics from ambulance work may affect 999 work.

Implications for society

- Are we happy to accept that we cannot see the health professional of our choice?
- No studies have been undertaken to test models to ensure efficiency or safety.

Answer 2

Mrs Patel, a 40-year-old lady you have not seen recently, attends with one of her children for a routine child health check. You notice she has several bruises at different stages. When you enquire about these, she is evasive. How would you proceed?

This problem demands tact and sensitivity to achieve a satisfactory outcome.

History

- Consider need for an interpreter and/or chaperone, perhaps from own ethnic or religious group, eg nurse or receptionist.
- Be aware of need for a good doctor–patient relationship, this may take time and several visits.
- Need to assure patient of confidentiality. Consider need to be discreet in record keeping as may attend in future with spouse or family.
- Is there a simple explanation for her bruises? A difficult child, a recent accident or clotting disorder. Need to approach the subject tactfully and offer opportunity to talk about her situation. Need to be respectful of her religion and society rules which may be different to your own. Is she alone? Women from the Indian subcontinent will often attend with either husband or family members and may not feel domestic violence is the business of the doctor.
- Are there any signs of depression? Any evidence of self-harm?
- Consider possibility that if abuse is occurring, it may be considered normal in her culture. Explore ideas, concerns and expectations if possible both of her role in home and your role. Why does she think she is being injured? Is the husband an alcoholic? Is she seeking a

role outside home or breaching accepted cultural norms, eg wants to get a job.

Management

- Offer advice on what she should expect from the medical and legal systems. Pursuing normal avenues employed in domestic violence may be inappropriate as she may not be prepared to risk family/ostracism from community.
- Suggest, if appropriate, seeking support from within community, eg priest or female relatives.
- If serious risk exists, encourage to seek legal assistance, eg from police.
- Offer information about support outside community, eg Samaritans.
- Consider seeking advice from MDU.
- Need meticulous note keeping in view of potential legal involvement.
- Consider PHCT meeting/significant event review. Any needs for organisation or individual, eg, greater cultural awareness. Are resources, eg leaflets/posters, available for victims of domestic abuse.

Wider management

- Is there a need for a local social worker from the patient's ethnic group?
- Is this an isolated problem or are there wider problems? Consider PCT-wide action, eg publicity campaign.

Answer 3

As a result of recent MRSA infections in your local community hospital, you are invited to sit on a committee looking into prevention of infection. You wish to make any protocol evidence based.

1 How would you ensure a comprehensive inclusion of data?

- Need to avoid inclusion bias. Decide on search strategy that is likely to answer the question while covering as much of the literature as possible.
- Ideally aim to include gold standard literature – double blind, randomised controlled studies published in peer-reviewed journals. Often impractical to search journals by hand (relies on local access to paper copies).
- Where quality RCT data do not exist, search for systematic reviews,

non-systematic reviews, case-control studies and case reports.

- Medline, Embase and Cochrane databases allow access to data from worldwide trials, without subscription, and are useful as a screening tool to identify studies for further consideration.
- Compendia of critical reviews such as *Bandolier* and *Clinical Evidence* allow readymade surveys of data.
- Drug company data may also be available, but those studies available are potentially susceptible to exclusion bias, ie trials with negative findings may be suppressed or not published.
- Internet searching may provide valuable data but suffers from the same problems as electronic databases as described above – plus the internet is unedited and some information is of dubious quality.
- Local knowledge, eg consultant microbiologists, public health teams may be useful as pointers to data, but need to beware influence of dogma and bias in current practice. Research may have been carried out locally or elsewhere that has not been published, and local experts may guide you to this.

2 **Comment on the strengths and weaknesses of the database search in reference material 1.1b**

Strengths

- Quick access to summarised data on millions of studies published worldwide in many languages
- Only includes published literature, mostly peer reviewed.
- Needs only a computer with internet access, so widely available.

Weaknesses

- Does not allow access to full papers. This can impede assessment of data for bias, since only limited data on methodology are available
- Critically dependent on quality of summary entered on to database.
- Only includes published literature.
- Cost of equipment to access data.
- Critically dependent on search methodology. Often requires training in efficient use.

3 **Discuss the data extraction methodology described in the Method**

Search strategy

- Developed in advance to search for relevant terms.
- Wide ranging databases to minimise language or cultural bias, eg includes publications in mandarin Chinese.

- Followed up with hand search of key journals but what is a hand search and what is a key journal? Potentially subjective and risks inclusion bias.

Study selection

- Full articles obtained if abstracts mention endemic or epidemic MRSA and an attempt at control in hospital. This allows first hand assessment of study methodology and results, but excludes data on control of non-epidemic or endemic MRSA.
- Prevention of MRSA transmission and infection is as important where it is rare as where it is common, particularly with regard to hygiene, so this may unnecessarily exclude some valid studies.
- The limitation to an element of prospective data collection is valid since retrospective data collection is prone to observer bias, however the policy on exclusion of retrospective data being applied only to some of the study settings (most intensive settings allowed) is illogical since these high cost settings are surely the ones where high quality evidence of efficacy is needed most to allow cost-effective use of resources.
- Exclusion of retrospective data would exclude, for example, a comparison of hospital A found to have low historical rates of infection with hospital B with high rates. Rejection of studies not mentioning an isolation policy is relevant to the study question but is prone to linguistic bias – there is no definition of isolation, so the selection criteria will only select those studies where the phrase 'isolation' is used, rather than, eg, 'segregation'.

Data extraction and synthesis

- Data was analysed to take into account statistical methodology and control for bias and confounders. The studies were then analysed independently by two reviewers.
- However, there is no mention of whether a consistent set of rules was used for this process and whether both reviewers examined all papers and then compared notes, and what steps were taken to resolve dispute. This information may be available elsewhere, but is important since this grading of data is crucial to the review process.

Answer 4

Data from the paper 'Isolation measures in the hospital management of methicillin resistant *Staphylococcus aureus* (MRSA): systematic review of the literature' (with copyright

permission from *British Medical Journal* 2004; 329: 533–539)
are given in reference material 1.1b and 1.1c.

1   Describe the problems associated with data quality in
    systematic reviews

- Systematic reviews rely on data that have been generated in the
  past. Problems with study design, confounders and bias cannot be
  controlled and pooling data tends to compound the problem by
  adding further sources of bias.
- Where data on outcomes are pooled and statistical data
  recalculated one particularly poor set of data arising out of a badly
  designed study may profoundly affect the result, particularly where
  small but potentially significant effects are being sought.
- Systematic reviews assume populations and interventions are
  comparable. Frequently this is not so. In the example of isolation
  nursing this may be single rooms in one hospital or complete
  isolation with barrier nursing in another. Similarly handwashing
  may be just soap and water or chlorhexidine/alcohol washing,
  which are not equivalent. Combining data from two such
  interventions may dilute any effects seen, good or bad.

2   With reference to table 3 (reference material 1.1b), comment
    on the studies included

- The studies that are felt to provide stronger evidence represent a
  mixture of settings, interventions and methodologies. They are
  based in a variety of settings from large teaching hospitals to a
  paediatric ICU with only 20 beds.
- Clearly the risks for cross infection are very different – a PICU will
  have dedicated staff who seldom see other patients and are
  geographically isolated within the hospital. Comparing this with
  large teaching hospitals where medical students among others may
  wander from ward to ward spreading infection is likely to bring in
  many potential confounders.
- Several of the studies introduce more than one intervention, eg
  Coello *et al* use single room isolation, nurse cohorting, contact
  screening, prompt discharge and active eradication of carriage.
  Other studies, eg Duckworth *et al* use mainly isolation. Clearly the
  interventions are not comparable and may disguise the true
  effective intervention.
- It is not clear what the outcomes are and how they are compared
  both within and between studies.
- To compare efficacy directly one needs a numerator, eg cases of
  MRSA and a denominator, eg patient admissions. It is not clear if
  any of the studies have attempted to quantify this.

- Trends in infection or colonisation with time may simply reflect changes in carriage in the general population or increased throughput of patients.

3   **With regard to your brief to implement an evidence-based strategy to reduce MRSA transmission in your local community hospital, what recommendations could you make from this evidence?**

Based on the data there appears to be limited evidence for any of the measures described. The data are of poor quality and multiple confounding influences exist which have not been controlled for. The evidence does suggest perhaps anecdotally that isolation and/or hygiene measures may reduce infections but clearly further evidence would be helpful. With regard to the community hospital setting none of the studies were carried out in such an environment so none of the results may be suitable for extrapolation to this environment. In the absence of firm evidence, the cost of any new measures needs to be considered before implementation of changes.

Answer 5

One of your partners announces that he wishes to become a GPwSI in ENT. What issues does this raise?

Issues for the practice

- The practice will inevitably lose clinical sessions and these will have to be replaced. This may be an opportunity to review working patterns, eg nurse practitioner or take on new staff, eg retainer.
- Money: Will the PCT pay for training costs (locum, course and exam fees) if not will the practice bear the expense? Will the pay for the work cover locum costs? If not, should the practice effectively subsidise the PCT, or should they pay for the partner to pursue his hobby?
- Benefits: Increased skills in ENT within the practice should reduce referrals and allow more effective treatment within the practice. It will also allow patients who would have been referred to a DGH to be seen at a local site with shorter waiting times.
- Potential benefits if practice is participating in devolved budgets/commissioning.
- If the practice has personal lists, increased time out of the practice will result in longer waits for appointments.
- Will patients who would otherwise have seen a consultant feel happy to see a GP?

Issues for the doctor

- Can he cope with pressures of study and time management that this will bring?
- Will his partners allow him sufficient time off work to study, or will he be expected to do it in his annual leave or on half days. This may spark resentment particularly if profits from GPwSI work are pooled.
- Will need support of primary care colleagues – they will need faith in him to refer.
- Why does he feel the need to expand into other areas? Is he bored, or does he have a genuine interest in ENT?

Issues for PCT

- Should facilitate referral management with alternatives to traditional referrals, reducing costs and freeing up more funds for other services.
- May allow use of under-utilised community hospital facilities.
- Will they pay for the training and running costs?
- May result in increased referrals as GPs with more experience pick up more problems in that area and refer more to secondary care.
- Will need to pay for equipment, eg nasoendoscope.

Issues for hospital

- How do hospital colleagues feel about patients being seen by GPs? Will this initiative damage relationships between primary and secondary care?
- Should allow hospitals to meet waiting times for outpatients.

Answer 6

Your next patient is a 58-year-old man who has had progressive weakness in his right leg. His EMG results have come back showing he has motor neurone disease. What issues would you aim to cover in the consultation?

Issues for the patient

Diagnosis

- Explain the likely diagnosis of motor neurone disease and how the diagnosis was made. Tailor explanation to patient, in terms of what they understand and what they want to know.
- Explore ideas concerns and expectations. What do they know about MND and its likely prognosis/treatment? Consider patient information leaflet to clarify issues raised.

- Be aware of awful reputation MND has and likely shock/bereavement reactions in patient and family. Be realistic but supportive. Allow plenty of time for questions now and at a later date. Avoid jargon.
- Offer second opinion if they wish.

Treatment

- What does the patient want?
- Explain treatment options: Riluzole may prolong life but not cure. Needs consultant referral to initiate treatment. Aim for effective symptom control, eg analgesia, baclofen for spasms.
- Involve PHCT as early as possible. Patient and family will need help with personal care, mobility and palliative care or district nurses. Speech therapy and dietician may be important later. Consider counselling for patient and family.
- Be prepared for questions about living wills/euthanasia that may arise.
- Advise re: support groups.

Issue for the family

- Consider their needs and what they can realistically be expected to do? Are they able to cope with caring at home, with support?
- Discuss with them the practice's system for dealing with carers, consent may be needed if information is to be passed to social services.
- Advice on disability living allowance eligibility and parking.
- Do they need genetic counselling? Do they want to know their risk?
- Involve OTs early if care is to be in the home.
- Is he the breadwinner? Loss of this role may have profound effects on his self-respect as well as financial effects on family unit.
- Any adaptations needed at home, eg stair lift, etc.

Issues for doctor

- Lengthy difficult consultation, likely to be emotionally draining. Consider a break for a cup of tea before the next patient.
- Any learning needs? Could he have been diagnosed earlier?
- Need to be accessible for patient, eg telephone queries and will need home visits.
- May find it difficult to break bad news. Consider training courses, eg run by palliative care teams.
- Patients may seek advice about areas that conflict with moral code, eg euthanasia.

Issues for society

- Ethical dilemma of prolonging life in terminal patient. Should euthanasia be allowed for such cases?
- Use of limited resources to fund expensive drugs that prolong life rather than providing palliative care resources, eg hospice nurses.

Answer 7

Please read the extract from 'Efficacy and safety of naltrexone and acamprosate in the treatment of alcohol dependence: a systematic review' (*Addiction* 2004; 99: 811–828, (*Bandolier* 126:3) given in reference material 1.2a and answer the questions below.

1   Comment on the style of data presentation chosen by the authors in Figure 1 of reference material 1.2b

- The data are presented as a L'Abbé plot.
- The effect of the intervention is plotted on the y-axis, the placebo on the x-axis. The line drawn x = y is the line of equal effect.
- Data above this line represent positive effect for the treatment, below represent positive effect for placebo.
- These charts are quick and easy to comprehend, and allow a visual representation of study size (diameter of circles) and allow rapid comparison of results in different trials (widely scattered circles = widely differing results)

2   What is your interpretation of the data in Figure 1?

- The data in Figure 1 suggest a positive effect for acamprosate in some studies for abstinence compared to placebo.
- The data are heterogeneous, however, and some of the studies, particularly the larger ones, cross the line of equality.
- The magnitude of the effect shows a dichotomous pattern with some of the studies suggesting abstinence rates of 35–45% and some 5–20%. This may reflect studies of different duration, eg one group of studies may show high abstinence at 4 weeks while another looks at abstinence at 1 year, with smaller effects seen.

3   What is your interpretation of the data in Figure 2?

- Figure 2 shows that the outcome, relapse, is associated more strongly with placebo than naltrexone, ie naltrexone is superior in preventing relapse.
- The studies are, however, generally small and diverse in magnitude of effect.
- The only large study crosses the line of equal effect, suggesting a

possibility of no benefit.

4   With regard to the data in Table 1 of reference material 1.2c, comment on the statement that 'Naltrexone is a safe and effective adjunct to the treatment of alcohol dependence'

- The data in Table 1 show a small effect in favour of abstinence and against relapse for naltrexone, however, the confidence intervals are wide and cross the line of no effect for abstinence.
- The number needed to treat is 10 to prevent relapse, ie 10 people have to be treated for one to benefit.
- The number needed to harm in terms of gastrointestinal events is 13, ie for every 13 patients treated 1 will suffer this side-effect, with similar rates for psychiatric events and discontinuation.[Q5] This suggests that patients are almost as likely to experience a side-effect as any benefit.
- In assessing the risk-benefit profile one would need more information on side-effects: if gastrointestinal side-effects included gastrointestinal bleeds this would suggest it is not likely to be a useful drug in treatment of alcohol dependence, if, however, side-effects were nothing more than flatulence it may be worth considering.

References

1 Efficacy and safety of naltrexone and acamprosate in the treatment of alcohol dependence: a systematic review. *Addiction* 2004; 99: 811–828
2 Outcomes for untreated individuals involved in randomized trials of alcohol treatment. *Journal of Substance Abuse Treatment* 2002; 23: 247–252

Answer 8

You are called in the middle of surgery by a mother who tells you that her 12-month-old daughter who has had a cold for the last couple of days is now having a fit. Describe how you would deal with this situation.

Immediate management

- Triage is vital in this situation. Accurate assessment of the situation is necessary to decide if an ambulance is more appropriate: Any history of previous seizures? Any rash? Any signs of meningitis? Any fever? Is the child breathing?
- Give first-aid advice on airway management. If able to attend

promptly do so; if not send ambulance. On arrival complete initial assessment. If still fitting consider rectal diazepam. If fever give rectal paracetamol and look for signs of cause, eg rash, chest signs, neck stiffness.

- Admit to paediatrics all first seizures, even when diagnosis is likely to be febrile seizure. This will reassure parents who probably have received the worst fright of their life. Expert assessment will ensure meningitis or brain tumours are not missed. If the history is suggestive of epilepsy they will need consultant assessment and treatment.
- Once patient has been admitted, reflect on situation: Any learning or skill needs? Are you competent in paediatric resuscitation? Any problems for patient accessing care? Were there any problems for patient talking to doctor? Review protocol for urgent visits.

Subsequent management

- Follow up patient with paediatricians to ensure you are aware of diagnosis.
- Offer to see parents soon to review and reassure about diagnosis.
- Explain management of future seizures. Provide rectal paracetamol and ensure family are prepared and competent to use. Consider patient leaflets. Ensure family are aware of how to access healthcare in emergency.
- Give plenty of opportunity for questions. There will be concerns over future health of child, possible brain damage, future activities, eg safe to swim, driving, etc. Parents may feel it is their fault, and may need reassurance. They may fear for future children and possible brain damage.
- Other carers, eg childminders may need similar advice and support.

Practice issues

- Any learning needs for practice team?
- Are staff aware of when to pass messages directly to doctor?

Answer 9

With regard to routine vaccinations, discuss recent developments in the following areas:

1   **5-in-1 vaccine for babies**

- This has been discussed in an editorial in the *British Medical Journal*[1].

- Pentavalent vaccine represents three changes to current vaccine regimen:
  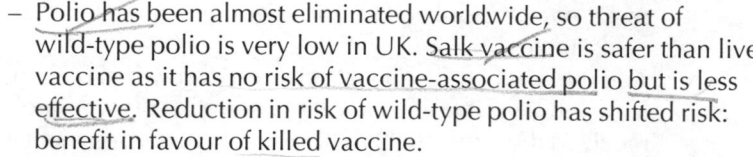
  - Polio has been almost eliminated worldwide, so threat of wild-type polio is very low in UK. Salk vaccine is safer than live vaccine as it has no risk of vaccine-associated polio but is less effective. Reduction in risk of wild-type polio has shifted risk:benefit in favour of killed vaccine.
  - Replacement of whole-cell pertussis vaccine with acellular vaccine is as effective as existing vaccine but has fewer side-effects such as fever and pain.
  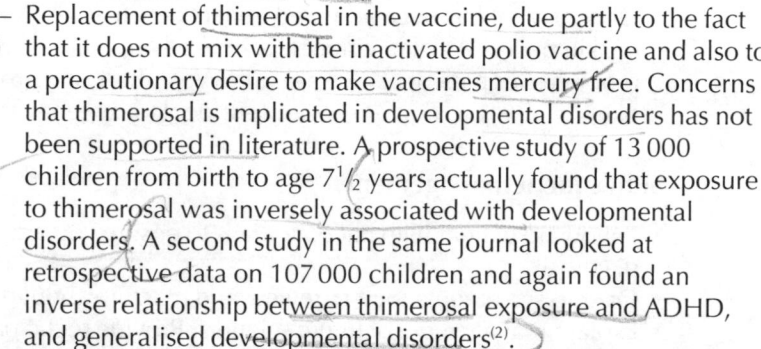
  - Replacement of thimerosal in the vaccine, due partly to the fact that it does not mix with the inactivated polio vaccine and also to a precautionary desire to make vaccines mercury free. Concerns that thimerosal is implicated in developmental disorders has not been supported in literature. A prospective study of 13 000 children from birth to age $7\frac{1}{2}$ years actually found that exposure to thimerosal was inversely associated with developmental disorders. A second study in the same journal looked at retrospective data on 107 000 children and again found an inverse relationship between thimerosal exposure and ADHD, and generalised developmental disorders[2].
- Some patient groups have expressed concern that the new vaccine will overload the immune system of their children. However, the switch to an acellular pertussis vaccine results in a reduction of almost 3000 antigens, while increasing the disease coverage[3].

2   **Indications for varicella vaccination and use of varicella immunoglobulin in the UK?**

- Guidance from Joint Committee on Vaccination and Immunisation[4] now recommends that all healthcare workers who have not had chicken pox or shingles at pre-employment assessment should have serological testing, with those who are negative being vaccinated.
- A study in the *British Medical Journal* in 2004[5] suggests that relying on history alone will miss seronegative subjects, particularly from the tropics, and suggests they should all have serological testing.
- The Green Book[4] suggests that susceptible contacts of immunocompromised individuals, eg close family members of child receiving chemotherapy, should be immunised.
- Use of varicella immunoglobulin is recommended for those patients who are at risk of severe infection (immunocompromised, pregnant and neonates) who are also not immune, and have had a significant exposure to varicella.

3 Construct an algorithm for the management of a pregnant woman exposed to chicken pox

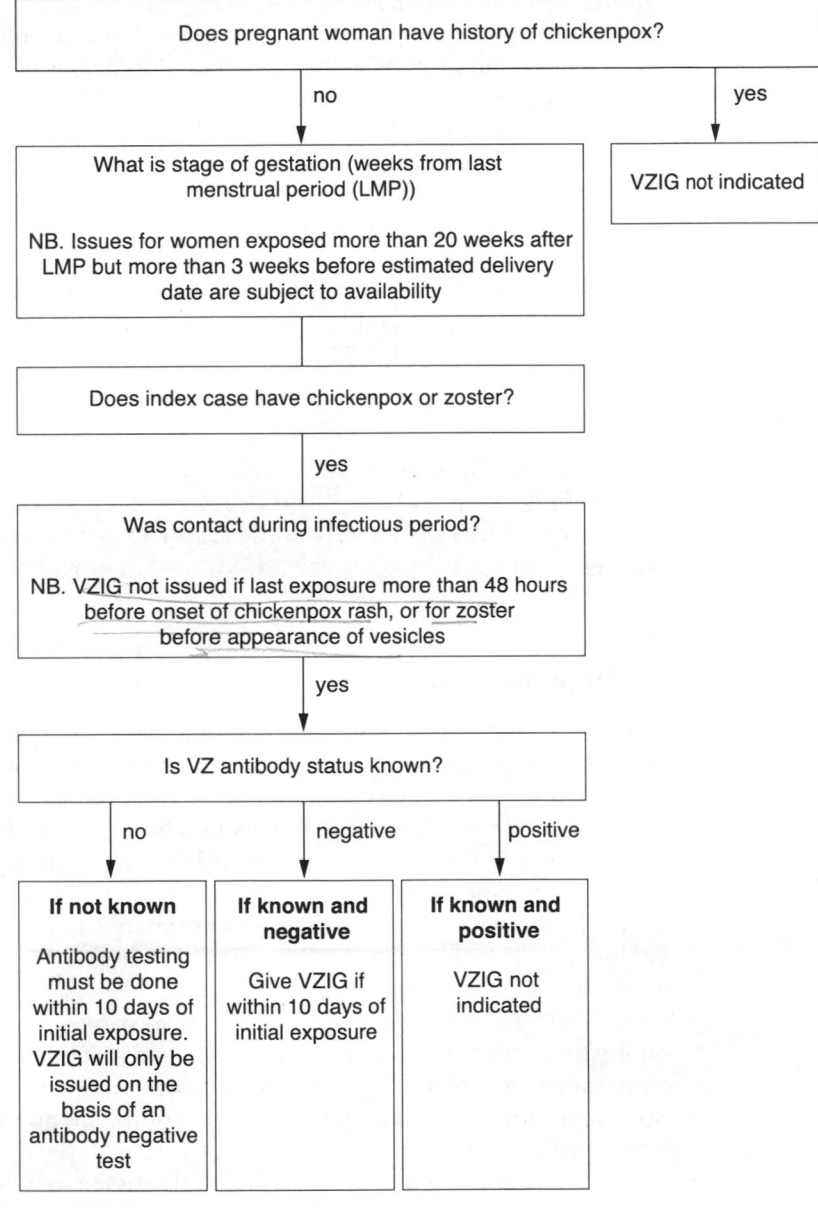

Does pregnant woman have history of chickenpox?

no

yes

What is stage of gestation (weeks from last menstrual period (LMP))

NB. Issues for women exposed more than 20 weeks after LMP but more than 3 weeks before estimated delivery date are subject to availability

VZIG not indicated

Does index case have chickenpox or zoster?

yes

Was contact during infectious period?

NB. VZIG not issued if last exposure more than 48 hours before onset of chickenpox rash, or for zoster before appearance of vesicles

yes

Is VZ antibody status known?

no

negative

positive

If not known

Antibody testing must be done within 10 days of initial exposure. VZIG will only be issued on the basis of an antibody negative test

If known and negative

Give VZIG if within 10 days of initial exposure

If known and positive

VZIG not indicated

References

1 Misconceptions about the new combination vaccine [editorial]. *British Medical Journal* 2004; 329: 411–412
2 Thimerosal exposure in infants and developmental disorders: a prospective cohort study in the United Kingdom does not support a causal association. *Pediatrics* 2004; 114: 577–583
3 Addressing parents' concerns: do multiple vaccines overwhelm or weaken the infants' immune system? *Paediatrics* 2002; 109: 124–129
4 www.dh.gov.uk/policyandguidance/healthandsocialcaretopics/ greenbook
5 Identification of potential candidates for varicella vaccination by history: questionnaire and seroprevalence study. *British Medical Journal* 2004; 329: 551–552

Answer 10

In an effort to reduce the cost of secondary referrals, your PCT proposes devolution of budgets to practice levels with the aim of encouraging practitioners to utilise alternative referral resources. Discuss the issues raised, for and against this proposal.

Issues for primary care

- Traditional options for the referring doctor are few, with little option other than referral to a consultant colleague. Devolution of budgets will encourage alternative providers to offer their services, eg specialist physio triaging orthopaedic referrals, use of incontinence specialist nurses to initiate assessment and management of patients prior to referral for surgery.
- This will encourage inward investment in primary care, eg employing assistants and specialist nurses, thus improving the range of facilities and services in the practice.
- Managing large budgets and the financial governance elements will require practices to take on more administrative staff before any savings are made, involving some financial risk to the practice.
- More appropriate skill mix, eg nurses seeing problems appropriate to their skills.
- Devolved budgets requires open and frank discussion of referral between doctors and agreement on common goals and strategies. Individuals may feel pressure to alter referrals against clinical judgement and may feel awkward having referrals discussed with colleagues.

- Referring practitioners must have confidence in the skills of the person they are referring to, or they will not use the service.
- Services are only worth developing where there is sufficient volume of referrals. Otherwise the running costs may exceed any savings made.

Issues for PCT

- Need to make a financial commitment to developing services, returns on training may not be made for many months or even years.
- May help to cap year on year growth in outpatient referrals, allowing investment elsewhere.
- Need to provide a financially attractive system that encourages practices to participate without devoting excessive sums to GPs profits.

Issues for hospital

- May allow them to meet access targets, eg by reducing inappropriate referrals.
- Significant diversion of income from secondary care to primary care or other providers may result in loss of services.
- May result in conflict between GP providers and consultants competing for patients.
- May need to provide better value for money, eg more patients seen by consultant rather than SHO.

Issues for patients

- May allow local provision of services, eg patients being treated in local practice or surgery.
- Patients may be treated more quickly, avoiding long waits.

Issues for society

- Are devolved budgets really rationing by the back door? Passing the rationing buck from politicians (who are widely distrusted) to GPs (who are widely trusted) may soften and disguise the blow.
- Do patients realise that the practice will effectively receive a financial incentive for referring or not referring them? If they find out, eg through the Freedom of Information Act, will it adversely affect the doctor–patient relationship?
- More effective use of resources will improve access to appropriate healthcare, eg incontinent ladies seeing a sympathetic local nurse rather than a distant consultant.

Answer 11

A local solicitor specialising in negligence claims writes to your practice offering £150 commission for every patient referred to him. What issues does this raise, and how would you respond?

This request raises a number of issues which must be considered before responding.

Issues for patients

- Patients who have been genuinely harmed but who are unlikely to receive large compensation payouts may be neglected by lawyers in favour of large payouts.
- Will there be any real benefit for them? If they have a genuine claim they should be able to launch a claim through a normal solicitor. Any likely payout will be reduced by the fee, and such solicitors often operate on a no win no fee basis. Typically any payout will see a large percentage going to solicitor.
- If they have been genuinely harmed, is resolution likely to be aided by a possibly lengthy court battle or would it be better aided by going through the patient advocacy service and to obtain an acknowledgement of their problems, explanation of circumstances and apology where appropriate.
- Risk of damaging relationships with doctors and other health professionals who may be guarded in their dealings with patients for fear of complaint. They may receive unnecessary investigations or treatments for fear of further complaint. This may expose to further risk, eg side-effects of operation or procedure.

Issues for doctors

- If accept commission for referral, this may be seen as tacit approval of the process. This may harm doctors' relationships with colleagues, particularly if they are subject of litigation.
- Need to declare financial interest. Patients may feel distrustful of their doctor's motives if they know the GP has a financial interest. May be seen less as the patients' advocate and more as looking after number one.
- Increasing litigation inevitably results in increased costs for the defence organisations resulting in increased subscriptions.
- Stress for person who is subject to complaint may ruin careers or even push people to suicide.

Issues for NHS

- Diversion of NHS funds from front-line services to pay compensation.

Issues for society

- Compensation culture constant threat to trust in services and financial burden on society.

Issues for legal profession

- May provoke distrust amongst doctors. In USA some sections of the medical profession are calling for blanket ban on treating litigation lawyers.
- Under Law Commission rule need to declare to client financial dealings with doctors.

Answer 12

It has come to your attention that your practice manager is spending increasing amounts of the working week 'working from home', the accounts are not up to date and several late reminders have arrived for unpaid bills. How would you approach the situation?

How has the situation arisen?

- Is the practice manager overworked? Rapid change in the NHS has led to a cascade of paperwork and it may be that they cannot keep up.
- Are they taking on extra work for other members of staff, eg computer work?
- Do they have issues outside work, eg relationship problems, that are affecting performance?
- Are there personality issues within the practice that make it an uncomfortable place for the practice manager to work?
- Is there any evidence of financial irregularity? Does the practice have robust systems to minimise fraud?

What must be done immediately?

- The problem should be addressed promptly. Failure to do so may cause further delay and increased pressure on the staff involved.
- The problem should be addressed tactfully, initially perhaps by the staff doctor as part of the appraisal process. This should be

non-confrontational and supportive and aim to identify the causes of the difficulties.
- The issues raised should be discussed by the partnership, who are ultimately responsible for the business. They need to decide if the issues raised are genuine and what action should be taken. If there is evidence of fraud, or serious underperformance any actions need to be in accordance with employment law.
- Financial irregularities should be discussed with the accountant.
- If the manager is over-worked, what can be done to address this? This may involve appropriate delegation, diversion of tasks or perhaps secretarial time for the manager.
- The partnership as employers owes a duty of care to the practice manager, and need to address any issues at work that are causing stress. Health and safety legislation covers stress and this may need to be addressed.
- If the practice manger is being bullied or there is conflict, this must also be addressed.
- Does the practice manager have unmet needs, eg IT or accountancy that need to be met say by the practice sending them on a course or sponsoring further qualifications in practice management.
- All outstanding debts should be paid.

What must be done in the future?

- Need to review financial governance. How did things get to this state? Need an outlet for staff to voice concerns ideally through an appraisal process. Is there a mentor system where staff can raise concerns?
- Is there a need to set up a local practice managers' group for mutual support and co-operation, eg with PCT audits, etc.
- Need to review how practice prioritises work.

Paper 2

Answer 1

A PCT audit of complaints in your locality shows that your practice received twice the average number of complaints compared with other practices. What issues does this raise?

Issues for the practice

- How did this arise? Review the inclusion criteria – is the practice correctly interpreting the audit criteria? Some practices may be under-reporting either deliberately or accidentally, by only including official complaints made in writing to the practice manager. Has the practice an open policy of encouraging complaints, verbal or written, no matter how trivial, in pursuit of perfection?
- What are the implications for the practice? Is it truly the worst practice in the area, and if so, why? Need to review the complaints, perhaps on a quarterly basis to allow reflection and change. This needs to be carried out with sensitivity and a no-blame culture where possible. Try to involve all affected team members wherever possible, and classify according to area, eg communication, clinical, organisational.
- Risks for the practice: Individual team members may feel threatened and discussion may end up becoming personal and destructive to the team. Team members may practise defensive medicine with excessive investigation and unnecessary treatment.
- What about good news? Does the practice or PCT record thanks, verbal or written and gifts?
- Are complaints about an individual a sign of burnout or stress?
- Appraisal – should include audit of significant complaints and how they are dealt with.

Issues for patients

- If the practice is substandard, patients may not be receiving adequate care. Patients who complain may be treated as troublemakers by team members.
- Patients may not have any way to express their feelings other than

complaints, eg unhappiness at appointment times may be expressed as a complaint since there is no other forum for discussion.
- Are patients at risk?
- Does the practice need a patients' forum or champion to represent them?

Issues for the PCT

- Is there really a broad spectrum of quality? If so the PCT should investigate as they now are the employer rather than the local health authority.
- Is the audit methodology robust? Review of case finding may reveal reasons for the disparity.
- The PCT must find a way to deal with serious complaints to protect the public without victimising individuals, to whom it owes a duty of care as an employer.

Issues for society

- Is this a reflection of our compensation culture? Are we too critical and demanding of public services and what will be the cost? Every pound spent on compensation is a pound less spent on services.

Answer 2

Mrs Smith, an 87-year-old widow is brought to see you by her daughter who is concerned that she may have Alzheimer's. How would you address the situation and what would be the aims of your management?

Assessment

- Acknowledge their concerns. What do they understand about Alzheimer's? What symptoms does she show? What is the patient's understanding of the situation? Any alternative explanation, eg infection, malnutrition?
- Review previous medical history/medication. Any history of cerebrovascular disease or other possible cause, eg syphilis in past, hydrocephalus?
- Perform mental state and physical examination. Further tests may be indicated, eg B_{12} and folate levels, FBC, thyroid function.
- Acknowledge ideas, concerns and expectations. Explain likely diagnosis and therapeutic options. Explain no treatment will reverse damage but some treatments may slow decline and potentially

improve quality of life.
- Offer written information and about support organisations. Offer early review to clarify issues raised and questions which may arise.
- If suitable and they wish to pursue active treatment, refer to psychiatrist specialising in dementia.

Management

- Social: Assess support networks and needs. Consider involving social services/CPN early to develop rapport. Remember needs of carers and consider registering carers. Consider respite needs. Are there daycare facilities available which may help to maintain social functioning?
- Financial: Apply for attendance allowance and disabled parking. May be eligible for council tax reduction.
- Medical: Gingko may reduce decline with an NNT of 7. It may cause bleeding however and care should be taken in patients on aspirin or other antiplatelet/anticoagulants.
- Anticholinesterase inhibitors reported in some studies to be effective in slowing decline and improving carer-rated quality of life. Needs consultant prescription and follow-up. Consider depression and treat accordingly.
- Offer regular follow-up and be accessible to carers. Consider power of attorney and living will if still mentally competent. Be prepared for time when family can no longer cope.

Answer 3

Concerning patient access to primary care services, comment on the advantages and disadvantages with regard to the different stakeholders involved.

Advantages

This was covered in a theme issue of the *British Journal of General Practice* (May 2004).

Government

- *NHS Plan* states that by end of 2004 everyone should be able to access a primary care professional within 24 hours and a doctor within 48 hours. Some politicians have staked reputations on this and seek to use extension of consumerism/choice to their political benefit. Faster access to a health professional often represented as increased access, which is thought to be a vote winner.

- Allows government to explore new models of primary care delivery which may be cheaper and reduce power of certain professional groups, eg doctors.
- Potential benefits through faster access in dealing with sickness absence faster, with quicker return to work.
- Potential increased efficiency of services through fewer missed appointments.
- A more fluid response to demand in theory will increase the capacity of primary care to deal with high-demand periods, eg flu epidemics, without overspill onto A&E departments.

Primary care trusts

- Opportunity to develop different models of care where appropriate, eg more use of community pharmacists, health visitors and district nurses to take strain off primary care.

Doctors

- Opportunity to re-evaluate working patterns and pass workload to other more appropriate staff, eg health visitor. Reduced DNAs and potential reduction in face-to-face consultations reported.

Practice staff

- More appointments to offer on the day reduces stress. Ability to triage calls.

Patients

- Able to obtain healthcare advice promptly at time of need. May value increased choice of provider, eg nurse rather than doctor.
- More consumer orientated. The public, after all, do bankroll the NHS.
- Increased choice of clinician possible, eg female doctor for gynaecological problems.

Disadvantages

Government

- In system without financial disincentives to seek advice, the loss of time disincentives may result in increased demand for trivia and need for more service provision rather than less.
- Increased medicalisation of normality and social problems if doctors are the most accessible point of help in society. May divert

workload away from more appropriate services, eg social services to primary care.

- Prescribing costs may increase if patients seen early in disease before it is evident whether disease is self-limiting or not.
- Financial: PCTs have to employ staff to facilitate process and fund implementation. Inevitably may result in loss of funds for other services.

Primary care trusts

- Yet more government targets to meet. Resources spent pursuing political goals at expense of less fashionable ones, eg mental health access.
- Diversion of work to pharmacists, health visitors and district nurses will increase their workload and costs. If they do not reduce GP appointments but simply delay them net cost will be increased.

Doctors

- Doctors value continuity of care and are often shown to be happier seeing their own patients than other doctors' patients. Studies of telephone triage show increased stress when not seeing patient face to face.
- More stress due to need to continuously monitor and satisfy demand, eg during flu epidemic may not be able to say 'No more'.
- May feel that the care they give is devalued by the notion that anyone will do.

Patients

- Less continuity of care may result in subtle, less evident, problems being missed in drive to deal with today's problems. Less opportunistic healthcare. More inconsistency of treatment, eg Dr A starts drug A for hypertension, then next time patient sees Dr B who changes to drug C.
- Patients with transport or telephone/communication problems, eg deafness may not be able to access services. Increased telephone traffic first thing in morning may make it impossible to get through until all suitable appointments are gone. May have difficulty arranging transport at short notice.
- Patients like ease of access, but place higher priority on doctor of choice. May lose this choice.
- Patients in certain occupations or schoolchildren may need to book in advance to arrange work commitments. Advanced Access may not allow this.

Staff

• Stress of manning telephone early in mornings when appointments are opened.

Answer 4

Mr Smith, a 78-year-old man, presents with symptoms of parkinsonism. How would you manage the situation?

Initial management

Diagnosis

• Review history and symptoms. Are they typical of parkinsonism? Consider alternative diagnoses.
• Examine neurologically with a view to confirming diagnosis/excluding other causes, eg essential tremor, alcohol withdrawal.
• Explore ideas, concerns and expectations. What does the patient think is the diagnosis? Why has he presented now? Family pressure? How is it affecting him? Inability to look after family or pursue interests? Expectations are important as Parkinson's disease has a bad public image despite effective treatments.
• Consider need for referral to confirm diagnosis either to convince patient, clarify diagnosis if clinical uncertainty or educate about the disease.
• Diagnosis may be a shock. Consider patient leaflet and offer review appointment to answer any questions.
Treatment
• Consider therapeutic treatments. Most patients treated with levodopa (Madopar) initially at low dose titrated according to response. If not tolerated consider ropinirole.
• Screen for depression, very common in Parkinson's. Treat where appropriate.
• Consider OT referral, eg raising chairs to maintain independence.
• Consider patient leaflet to reinforce advice regarding treatment and prognosis. Advise on support groups.
• Look at effects on family – is he a carer? Does he need benefits or disabled parking sticker?

Ongoing management

• Regular review initially to support through initial phase of treatment, and deal with questions and problems as they arise.

- Consider needs of family, eg concerns about genetic susceptibility, ability to self-care and long-term prognosis.

Other areas of management

- Is there a need for a patients' group/expert patient programme in the area? May allow peer support and empower patients.
- Is there a need for greater public understanding of Parkinson's disease? Many patients go undetected because they don't realise they have a problem.
- Any learning needs for doctor or team?

Answer 5

MRSA is an increasing problem in all aspects of healthcare. Discuss strategies for preventing and treating infection with respect to the current literature.

Prevention of infection

- A systematic review in the *British Medical Journal* in 2004[1] found many of the studies were of poor quality, but that isolation may reduce transmission even in endemic situations. Isolation techniques included isolation wards, single-bedded rooms and barrier precautions.
- A small observational study of soap use in general practice found large variations in soap consumption suggesting large variation in handwashing practice[2], and strenuous efforts to enforce and encourage handwashing by staff have been unable to get this above 60–70% take up[3].
- The DOH has introduced *The Matron's Charter* (www.doh.gov) that will seek to establish a cleanliness culture across the NHS, with infection-control training for all staff, matrons having overall control over cleaning with the power to withhold payment to contractors.
- Enforcement of infection-control policies is also achieved through the Commission for Health Audit and Inspection, which includes hygiene when assessing hospital performance.
- Surveillance of infections in hospital found that rates were higher in teaching hospitals and particularly associated with devices such as central lines. It has been suggested that surveillance should be targeted at these high-risk cases.
- The rates of nosocomial infection in Britain are similar to those in other countries in Europe, but a much larger proportion of these are MRSA – 42% of bacteraemias were MRSA in the year 2000. Data from systematic reviews suggest that rigid isolation and hygiene

measures can reduce infection even in endemic areas[3].

• Successful control strategies have been developed in the USA and the Netherlands using a search and destroy method, based on screening staff and patients, particularly in high-risk areas such as the ICU and hospital transfers[4,5].

• MRSA is becoming a problem in the community with outbreaks reported in prisons and other sites. These do not seem to be exported from hospital, but arise in the community. Circumstances where susceptible individuals live in close proximity to each other, eg nursing homes, are particularly at risk of infection brought from hospital on patient discharge[3].

An editorial in the *British Medical Journal* in 2003[6] suggested that multidrug resistant MRSA may be acquiring sensitivity to older antibiotics such as co-trimoxazole, but pointed out that the human factor, ie antibiotic-prescribing patterns, is critical in both acquisition of resistance and its loss in later generations.

References

1 Isolation measures in the hospital management of methicillin resistant *Staphylococcus aureus* (MRSA): systematic review of the literature. *British Medical Journal* 2004; 329: 533–539

2 Audit of soap usage by a primary care team.*British Medical Journal* 2003; 327: 1453–1454

3 Controlling methicillin resistant *Staphylococcus aureus*. *British Medical Journal* 2003; 327: 1177–1178

4 A Dutch approach to methicillin resistant *Staphylococcus aureus*. *European Journal of Clinical Microbiology and Infectious Diseases* 1999; 18: 461–466

5 SHEA guideline for preventing nosocomial transmission of multidrug resistant strains of *Staphylococcus aureus* and *Enterococcus. Infection Control and Hospital Epidemiology* 2003; 24: 362–386

6 Old drugs for new bugs [editorial]. *British Medical Journal* 2003; 326: 235–236

7 Device-related sources of bacteraemia in English hospitals – opportunities for the prevention of hospital-acquired bacteraemia (*Journal of Hospital Infection* 2003:53;46–57)

Answer 6

Read the extract in reference material 2.1 from the paper 'Long term donepezil treatment in 565 patients with Alzheimer's disease (AD2000): randomised double blind trial. AD2000 Collaborative Group.' (with copyright permission from *The Lancet* 2004; 363: 9427) and answer the questions below.

1   Comment on the study population, study design and outcomes

- The study population is appropriate for this study since it represents the patient group for whom donepezil is licensed and are the ones who stand to gain the most from any intervention by maintaining independence.
- The study is reasonably large so should provide sufficient power. The study is a randomised double blind placebo controlled trial which is the gold standard for assessing the impact of an intervention. This should minimise observer bias.
- Outcomes are both clinically appropriate and objective, using validated scales, although entry to institutional care may have possible influences, not directly related to need, such as resource availability, ability of carers to cope in the home, financial support. However, this outcome is relevant as the study is looking at cost vs benefit for the intervention.

2   Comment on the relevant data under the following headings:

Patients

- The data shows a statistically significant benefit for patients in terms of MMSE test score decline and functionality.
- The confidence intervals and p values <0.05 both suggest this is a genuine effect.
- The intervention was also shown to be safe, with no increase in adverse events or deaths between control and intervention.
- No attempt was made to assess quality of life.

Carers

- There were no significant differences in carer psychopathology or unpaid time.
- No attempt was made to quantify carers' quality of life, which may be significant in assessing benefits.
- There was no statistically significant difference in progression of disability or entering care, although for both of these a small benefit was seen.
- Larger or longer studies may provide a better estimate of whether this is a true effect, since the confidence intervals are wide.

Society

- Donepezil does not seem to provide a cost-effective method of reducing the financial burden of Alzheimer's on individuals or society, since it does not significantly reduce admissions to care homes, caregiver time or care costs.

Answer 7

The Quality and Outcomes Framework of the new GMS contract presents many new obstacles. Discuss the likely challenges and how these can be overcome.

For doctors

- Sense of scrutiny: Payment will be by results and may cause problems between partners where one person is perceived to be not pulling weight. Quality and Outcomes Framework assessment visits will place practice in spotlight and may be a difficult cultural change.
- Need to practise evidence-based medicine. Some doctors feel general practice is an art and cannot be described in numbers and codes. Patients may be lost in the search for points, with their personal medical needs neglected as we pursue public health aims of new contract.
- Need to be competent in use of IT to do the work and to prove it has been done.
- Need to address learning needs both clinically and in IT. Do individuals have special skills, eg in diabetes, that will help practice reach goals.
- Need to be realistic about aspirations.
- Consider skill mix: Better to employ nurses for chronic disease management? Phlebotomist to free up nursing time?

For staff

- Need robust recall systems to ensure patients are called in for treatment.
- Audit of progress towards aspiration needs to be carried out regularly to guide work.
- Consider special clinics for GMS work to ensure sufficient appointments are available to prevent chronic disease management being squeezed out by acute problems.
- Plan workload according to resources, eg aim to do bulk of work outside summer holidays/flu epidemics.
- Consider systems for collecting data, eg opportunistic recording of smoking status, etc., as well as formal chronic disease sessions.
- Staff must understand role of points. Consider performance-related

pay to involve whole team – everyone is needed to make the system work and involvement in reward will ensure participation.
• Need training in coding, etc.

For patients

• Personal vs public health needs. The interventions in the contract are public health based and many patients will not notice any difference to their health other than taking a lot more pills.
• Polypharmacy as we chase targets. Risk of iatrogenic illness, eg gastrointestinal bleed on aspirin.
• Their individual problems may be lost in drive to collect points.
• May find it difficult to get routine appointments as appointments are diverted to chronic diseases.
• Patients with chronic diseases not included in the Quality and Outcomes Framework, eg Parkinson's disease or rheumatoid arthritis may be neglected.

For PCTs/hospitals

• Drug costs are likely to rise sharply with opportunity cost, eg elective surgery.
• Echocardiograms – urgent cases may be delayed due to referrals for non-urgent patients referred only to meet points.
• Can PCTs afford to pay the points? Government estimated originally 750 points per practice and budgeted accordingly. In some areas the likely points total may be much higher.

Answer 8

A 43-year-old man with a history of chronic backache presents with a 3-day history of lumbar backache with radiation to the right leg. Discuss his management with reference to the literature.

Acute presentation

• Review symptoms: Triage via RCGP guidelines[1]. Describe red flag symptoms (weight loss, fever, weight loss, perineal anaesthesia or bladder/bowel dysfunction, progressive nature, significant previous medical history, eg tuberculosis, cancer) which may herald significant pathology. If there is any suggestion of acute cord compression refer immediately.
• Examination: Neurological examination should include sensory, motor and reflexes, straight leg raising, look for evidence of

significant cord injury, eg sensory level, saddle anaesthesia. Look out for evidence of systemic illness, eg cancer.
- Management: If red flag symptoms or signs are present refer urgently to specialist. If indicated, eg possible wedge fracture, consider use of X-ray although for uncomplicated lumbar backache this has not been shown to affect outcome[2].
- If red flags not present, offer explanation, reassurance and offer treatment advice. Stay active, simple analgesia/anti-inflammatories where no contraindications exist. Try to avoid potentially addictive treatments for management of potentially chronic problems.
- Encourage early return to work.
- Follow up advice with patient information leaflets if appropriate. Consider use of physio or osteopath/chiropractor. Data suggest little difference in long term outcomes between either of these. A study in the *British Medical Journal* in 2004[3] compared outcome between simple advice from physio and 6-week course of intensive physio and found no difference in outcome.

Long-term management

- Risk of long-term disability may be predicted by 'yellow flags'[4], psychosocial markers of potential chronicity, eg social or financial problems, depression, low self esteem and job satisfaction, fear, avoidance and negative attitudes about backache. A systematic review in the *British Medical Journal* in 2003[5] found 80% had returned to work within one month, but that 73% patients had at least one recurrence in the next 12 months.
- Be aware of risk of depression as a cause and consequence of backache. Avoid stigmatising patients. Encourage lifestyle changes to promote healthy living, eg smoking, exercise, etc.
- Review social situation. Is he incapable of work? Consider all work test if prolonged sick certification. Is there any gain from the sick role? Exempt from work/home duties.
- Consider effect on family, loss of self-esteem and breadwinner.
- If chronic, be open to request for second opinion and consider referral if surgery an option.
- If large numbers of patients with back pain in practice area consider back classes, eg run by physios to promote healthy attitude to back pain and treatment/prevention, and provide support.

References

1 *Clinical guidelines for management of acute low back pain.* London: Royal College of General Practitioners, 1996
2 Radiography of the lumbar spine in primary care patients with low

back pain: randomised controlled trial. *British Medical Journal* 2001: 322; 400–405

3 Randomised controlled trial of physiotherapy compared with advice for low back pain. *British Medical Journal* 2004; 329: 708

4 Guide to assessing psychosocial yellow flags in acute low back pain: risk factors for long term disability and work loss. Wellington, New Zealand. Accident Rehabilitation and Compensation Corporation of New Zealand, 1997

5 Acute low back pain: systematic review of prognosis. *British Medical Journal* 2003; 327: 323

Answer 9

In the capacity of team doctor to a local football team you are asked to give advice on physical conditioning and training, specifically to reduce the risk of injuries during training. In an attempt to make any advice evidence based, you research the literature and come across a paper (reference material 2.2a) entitled 'Effects of stretching before and after exercising on muscle soreness and injury: systematic review' (with copyright permission of the *British Medical Journal* 2002; 325: 468–70).

1 What problems might be encountered when conducting a systematic review of this area?

For data to be compared in a systematic review, the outcome measures need to aim for similar populations of subjects, with demographic features in common, with standardised interventions and standardised outcomes.

- Problems that might be expected include heterogeneity of subjects – physical conditioning and prevention of injury is important in almost all sports and in many occupational fields such as the military and fire service. The subjects are therefore likely to be very different, eg one study may look at army recruits on forced marches in army boots while another looks at elite female netball players. Data from one group is unlikely to be comparable with that from the another.
- Interventions to prevent the outcome are difficult to standardise even within studies – What is a standard stretch? How long for? Which muscle groups?
- This may be improved through group stretching with a leader following a protocol, but there is still likely to be significant interpersonal variation in extent of stretching. Randomisation is easy, but having control groups is not. Some studies may have no warm up as a control, others a warm up without stretching. Can

these two studies be compared?

- Confounders may influence the apparent results at the outcome level. The aetiology of sports injury is multifactorial: despite the best warm-up an athlete may trip over a loose stone and injure themselves.
- The likelihood of an injury is higher the harder athletes push themselves, and serious athletes are more likely to follow a rigorous warm-up, so it may appear that a rigorous warm-up is more likely to produce injury.
- Outcomes are subjective. How is muscle soreness quantified? Using a Likert scale may allow comparison, but is very subjective and prone to recall bias. Use of specific injuries is also sport specific and dependent on technique.

2   **Comment on the data in Figure 1 of reference material 2.2b**

- The data for 24, 48 and 72 hours show a consistency across the five studies with a range of results crossing the line of no effect.
- The pooled effects are all close to 0 with the pooled data at each time interval crossing zero. This suggests the intervention is unlikely to be significantly superior to the control.
- The confidence intervals are narrow, suggesting the true results do indeed lie around zero, and larger studies are unlikely to show an effect.

3   **Comment on the data in Figure 2 of reference material 2.2b**

Figure 2 shows survival curves for two studies.
- These show that the number of subjects who reach the endpoint (being injury free) progressively decreases in both the control and intervention groups for both studies, with very close survival curves for each intervention and its corresponding control.
- The overall survival for both control and intervention groups in Pope et al 1998 is greater than in Pope et al 2000.
- This does not mean that the intervention in Pope et al 1998 was any better than the intervention in Pope et al 2000, since they are different studies and may not be similar in terms of subjects, setting, intervention or outcomes. The data suggest that the intervention in either study was not significantly better than control at preventing injury.

4   **What advice would you give to your team coach as a result of reading this data?**

Based on the data in Figures 1 and 2, there is no apparent difference in either muscle soreness or likelihood of injury in subjects who stretch before exercise and controls.

Answer 10

> As part of a prescribing review, it is apparent that prescriptions for COX 2 inhibitors are increasing rapidly. One of your partners seems to be responsible for much of this, which she justifies by arguing that money spent on drugs is more than saved on admissions for gastrointestinal bleeds. You agree to look into this.

1   How would you go about researching this topic?

- Need to gather data on cost-effectiveness vs side-effect profile.
- Search literature for data relating to efficacy compared with usual treatment, then relate this to cost.
- Ideally data would be from systematic reviews, meta-analysis or double-blind RCT to remove placebo effect, and preferably head to head study with groups matched for demographic and disease characteristics.
- Studies on side-effect profile should again be blinded to remove reporting bias, with defined clinically relevant outcomes, eg endoscopic proven gastrointestinal bleed rather than surrogate outcomes (anaemia or FBC).
- Account of non-gastrointestinal side-effects should also be made in studies.
- Studies should include where possible data on drop-outs, and studies should be on an intention-to-treat basis to be strictly applicable to everyday clinical practice.

2   What important considerations should be taken when assessing a new treatment for a condition?

- Is it safe? An arthritis drug that takes the pain away but causes you to die of a heart attack is of little practical benefit.
- Does it interact with other medications? Eg can it be taken with warfarin?
- Does it work? If so, is it significantly better than other treatments?
- How expensive is it compared with other drugs for similar treatments? Drugs with marginal clinical benefits that are much more expensive than alternatives may have significant effects on resources available for other treatments, eg hydrotherapy services, physio.

Consider the extract in reference material 2.3 from the paper 'Comparison of lumiracoxib with naproxen and ibuprofen in the Therapeutic Arthritis Research and Gastrointestinal Event Trial (TARGET), reduction in ulcer complications: randomised controlled trial' (with copyright permission from *The Lancet* 2004; 364: 665–674). With regard to the results, calculate the following data:

3   R]elative risk reduction for lumiracoxib vs NSAIDs in patients not taking aspirin

- Relative risk reduction = risk in NSAID group/risk in lumiracoxib group
- RRR = 100% × 1.09/0.25 = 436%

4   Absolute risk reduction for lumiracoxib vs NSAIDs in patients not taking aspirin

- Absolute risk reduction = risk in NSAID group – risk in lumiracoxib group
- ARR = 1.09 – 0.25 = 0.84%

5   Number needed to treat with lumiracoxib instead of NSAID to prevent one case of complications, in patients not taking aspirin

- Number needed to treat = 100/ARR
- NNT = 100/0.84 = 119

6   Number needed to harm for patients taking NSAIDs without aspirin

- Number needed to harm = 100/risk in intervention group
- NNH = 100/1.09 = 91.7

7   Assuming that lumiracoxib costs £15 per patient per month, while conventional NSAIDs cost £3 per month, comment on the suggestion that COX 2s offer significant overall savings when cost of treating gastrointestinal complications is considered.

- Number needed to treat to prevent one upper gastrointestinal bleed using lumiracoxib rather than conventional NSAID = 119
- Cost of treating 1 person for 1 year with lumiracoxib rather than NSAID = 12 × (cost of lumiracoxib – cost of NSAID) = 12 × 12 = £144
- Total cost of prescribing lumiracoxib to prevent 1 gastrointestinal bleed = 119 × 144 = £17 136

- This would seem to be rather more than the cost of treating 1 episode of upper gastrointestinal bleed with endoscopy and in-patient stay.

Answer 11

Your next patient is a 33-year-old man who works in a local factory. He tells you he had diarrhoea for three days, which has now settled, but that he needs a sick note for work. How would you approach the situation?

The following issues need to be considered when dealing with the request.

Why does he want a sick note?

- Is illness genuine? Does he have a poor sick record and is he at risk of disciplinary action? Patients with poor sick records may have genuine illness, eg ulcerative colitis and need frequent time off. They may be discriminated against.
- Have there been previous episodes of absenteeism and requests for sick notes?
- Are there any other problems, eg alcohol or drug abuse, that may account for his behaviour?
- Is there a problem at work, eg bullying, that he is avoiding? He may not feel able to admit this depending on his cultural beliefs.
- Does he have family problems? Is diarrhoea an excuse for depression. May not be able to admit depression.
- What are his ideas, concerns and expectations? He wants a sick note and expects one. Is he aware that sick note rules have changed and that he may self-certify for the first week?
- Are his employers refusing to accept self-certification, insisting on doctor's notes?
- May be hostile to suggestion that he does not need a sick note. He may feel doctor's suggestion that he does not need a sick note is because the doctor does not believe illness is genuine.

Management of immediate situation

- Discuss illness and tactfully enquire about the symptoms and any associated problems.
- Enquire why he didn't seek help when ill. Was it over the weekend when normal GP was unavailable?
- Ask why he feels he needs a sick note when law states that all employees may self-certify for first week of illness. Explain that sick notes should not be pre-dated and should not be used when illness

has passed with resolution of symptoms.
- Explain the self-certification system.
- Try to encourage him to use self-certification. Failure to do so will reinforce this pattern of health-seeking behaviour.
- If employer is insisting on a sick note, explain that the employer should normally bear the cost of a private sick note.
- If patient is hostile, consider giving sick note to avoid confrontation.

Management of future problems

- Review with receptionists. Consider getting a supply of self-certification forms and explanatory notes for both patients and employers to hand out rather than use GP appointments inappropriately.
- Is everyone aware of sick note rules?
- Ensure consistency among team. If one GP is giving out sick notes easily this may undermine efforts by others.
- Is there a problem with a local employer? If so consider a letter to the personnel department to explain the rules.
- If practice is going to charge for private sick notes, check with local practices to ensure consistency.

Answer 12

You are interrupted in the middle of surgery by one of your nurses who has been doing the baby clinic. She has discovered that the last patient, a 18-month-old girl, received a meningitis C vaccination instead of MMR. What issues does this raise and how would you react?

Issues for the patient

- Is the patient at risk? The patient has received an unnecessary vaccination at the expense of a necessary one, and will thus be at risk of measles, mumps and rubella until vaccinated. In this case, in the absence of allergy, the patient is unlikely to suffer much more than some local swelling.
- The parent's confidence in the practice, nurse and vaccination may be damaged and this may result in reduced uptake of vaccinations in future.

Issues for the nurse

- Loss of confidence in abilities may affect other areas of work, resulting in reduced efficiency.
- Are there any learning needs? Why did she give the wrong

vaccination? Was it ignorance or incompetence?
- Is she appropriately trained for the role? Does she understand the vaccination schedule?
- Is she under pressure and cutting corners?

Issues for the practice

- Need to be prepared for anger and possible complaint. Deal with this according to practice policy.
- Need to review protocols for vaccination storage and administration/checking.

Management of the situation

- Check the facts, eg telephone public health consultant regarding possible risk to patient.
- Someone needs to visit the family and explain the situation as soon as possible. This should be someone the family trusts, ideally the registered GP.
- Honest explanation of what happened and why, what the effects are likely to be and what must be done now.
- Offer opportunity to see someone again soon to discuss any issues they wish to raise.
- Need to discuss the incident at next significant event meeting and agree change to prevent recurrence.
- Advise the family of the outcome of the meeting and what has been done to prevent recurrence.

Paper 3

Answer 1

See reference material 3.1a, part of a paper entitled 'Meta-analysis of increased dose of inhaled steroid or addition of salmeterol in symptomatic asthma (MIASMA)' (with copyright permission from *British Medical Journal* 2000; 320: 1368–1373).

1 Comment on the outcome measures used

The outcome measures mentioned in the abstract are clinically relevant but imprecise. What is efficacy? Is it objective changes in peak flow or FEV or in the subjective symptoms?

2 Comment on the methods for identifying suitable studies

- The researchers searched EMBASE, Medline and GlaxoWellcome databases, considering all studies in any language.
- Study search and selection was conducted by one person in isolation. Explicit criteria were used in the search. There is no mention in the methods of independent verification of screening, which may allow inclusion bias.
- All the studies included were sponsored by GlaxoWellcome. This may be coincidence, or may represent inclusion bias.
- Including the GlaxoWellcome database may remove publication bias if all clinical trials, ie including those that failed to show a significant effect, are represented. If, however, the database is selective it may introduce more bias. The GlaxoWellcome database is not externally reviewed, so we cannot know whether it is free from bias.
- The screening flow chart shows that the process of screening was relevant to the clinical question, ie comparing increased steroid to salmeterol.

3 Comment on the studies included

- The review suggests that it is looking at the question of increasing inhaled steroids from 100 to 400 µg of beclomethasone (50 to 200 µg of fluticasone) or adding salmeterol (step 3 of asthma guidelines, The British Guidelines on Asthma Management *Thorax*

1997; 52(Suppl 1); 51–52). The studies included, however, had a range of inhaled steroid doses from 200 to 1600 µg per day. Are these patients comparable, since they may represent very different groups of asthma patients, some of whom may not be at step 3 of the asthma protocol or equivalent?

- Separate analysis of groups by steroid type and dose may show whether there is a steroid-specific effect confounding the results.
- The studies are all large, which gives the systematic review sufficient power when they are pooled.

4   Comment on the results shown in Table 5 of reference material 3.1b

- The results of all the individual studies fail to show a benefit for salmeterol compared with increased steroids. Pooled results appear to show a small benefit for salmeterol, but the confidence intervals are wide and they approach the line of no effect. The p values given (0.79 and 0.85) are not statistically significant.
- The treatment effect is 2.73%, ie a number needed to treat (NNT) of 37.

5   Comment on the applicability of these results to clinical practice

These results fail to show any significant difference between the two therapeutic choices. Although this may not show that salmeterol is better, it does not show that it is worse. Steroids are not without side-effects and it may be that salmeterol is a better choice at stage 3 of the asthma guidelines if it produces the same clinical effect with fewer side-effects.

Answer 2

An 18-year-old model comes to you complaining of a 3-month history of amenorrhoea.

Outline your management

Amenorrhoea is a common problem, but in this consultation it is important to be empathic and ensure the patient feels listened to, with her concerns taken seriously.

History

- Take full medical, menstrual and sexual history.
- Is she pregnant or using contraception?
- Any prescribed or illicit drug use, eg Depo-Provera, phenothiazines,

amphetamines?

- What are her concerns/ understanding of the problem – worried about pregnancy/STDs/infertility/gynaecological disease?
- Why has she presented now – does a friend or family member have gynaecological or fertility problems? Any relationship difficulties?
- Explore psychological issues, eg career pressures to maintain ideal weight or image causing eating disorders. Look for weight changes and purging or laxative abuse. The patient may resent questioning. Is she depressed? Is she happy in her job? Is she being sexually exploited?

Examination/investigations

- Any evidence of excessive weight loss – BMI, lanugo hair, skin changes, electrolyte disturbance.
- Consider pregnancy and blood tests – usually after six months of amenorrhoea but if patient or doctor need reassurance, or there is suspicion from the history, check prolactin, LH/FSH, oestradiol, testosterone, TFTs.

Management

- Advise her about ideal weight, healthy eating habits, risks of excess weight loss.
- If she is pregnant, offer all options and support.
- This is an opportunity to discuss contraception. Tailor efficacy/side-effects to lifestyle, eg avoid acne/weight gain with Depo-Provera. She may be happy not to have periods but you need to ensure she understands the need for contraception.
- Consider gynaecological referral if you suspect any abnormality. Consider osteoporosis prevention if there is prolonged oestrogen deficiency.
- If there is an eating disorder or psychological illness, consider referral to counsellor, CPN or specialist eating disorder service. Tailor treatment plan to lifestyle, eg psychotherapy may not fit in with travel and she may not engage.

Issues for the doctor

- Potentially long, difficult consultation that may overrun. Consider review appointments.
- Potential awkwardness for male GP seeing attractive female patients; may feel more comfortable handing over to female colleague. How does the patient feel?
- Your own attitude to glamour industry may affect feelings – do you

see it as exploitation? Do you have teenagers of your own with concerns about eating disorders?
- A patient who is pregnant and requesting abortion may cause ethical difficulties for the doctor.
- Any educational needs regarding amenorrhoea and eating disorders?

Wider issues

- Eating disorders are increasingly prevalent. Be aware of signs to allow early identification and help.
- Need to educate PHCT. Consider literature or posters in practice, highlighting the problem and how to seek help.
- Need to lobby nationally against portrayal of thin as 'ideal' by the media and glamour industry.
- Improve provision of services for those with eating disorders – currently very patchy.

Answer 3

The father of an 8-year-old girl requests that you record and investigate his concerns that his estranged wife may have Munchausen's-by-proxy. What are the implications of this?

This situation encompasses a number of difficult issues and the response to the request needs to be carefully considered. The implications can be categorised in the following way.

Implications for the child

- Is she at risk?
- What would be the effect of bringing allegations out in the open? Will parental access be denied, exacerbating the emotional trauma of divorce? Will the child be subjected to unpleasant investigation to confirm or deny illness?
- What would be the emotional effect on the child of being used as a pawn?
- Genuine childhood illness may be untreated either because of the suspicion that her mother is fabricating symptoms, or because the mother fears being accused of fabricating illness.
- Who should consent to investigations on child to prove or disprove allegations?

Implications for the father

- May be hostile if he feels he is ignored, may be worried about his

children but feel unable to act.
- May be looking for evidence for custody battle.

Implications for the mother

- Will need support and advice, whether or not allegations are true.
- Is the father trying to obtain confidential information about her?
- Genuine psychological problem may have been neglected.
- If the allegations are untrue, stigma may persist, resulting in considerable social problems, eg work.
- Investigating the allegations may cause a breakdown in relationship with the GP or health visitor.

Implications for the GP

- Very difficult case; you will need to be aware of your feelings and emotional state, eg fear of missed diagnosis.
- Is there an educational need? Review knowledge of Munchausen's.
- May be at risk of accusations of breach of confidentiality if reveals medical records of wife or daughter to father, or negligence if allegations are ignored but are true.
- Potential conflict of interest if you are also the mother's GP. Can you avoid taking sides?
- Consider need for medico-legal advice, eg from MDU.

Implications for the PHCT

- Health visitor may have a better relationship with mother than GP, although this may be a hindrance.
- Discuss with PHCT to ensure everyone is aware of allegations, and has a chance to air their thoughts.
- Do other members of the PHCT share concerns? If so, why have they failed to mention them before? Do they feel unable to air them?
- Good relations with social services to ensure appropriate organised and measured response.
- Is there an educational need for PHCT? Significant event meeting?
- Need to ensure everyone is aware of confidentiality issues.

Implications for secondary care

- May require paediatric or psychiatric input.

Answer 4

Mrs Bhatia is having hospital-initiated infertility treatment and attends for a repeat script. You note you wrongly prescribed her clomipramine last time instead of clomiphene. What issues does this raise?

Such incidents rarely happen in isolation. Investigating the accident chain allows us to install safeguards to prevent recurrence.

Consultation issues

- Acknowledge guilt and embarrassment about the mistake.
- Avoid temptation to ignore incident and shrug responsibility.
- You need to be open and give a full apology to the patient and her partner (if present).
- The consultation may be long; consider a double appointment.
- Allow and encourage the patient to ask questions about what has happened. She may need to be offered more time at a later date.
- Be aware of language problems in explaining the mistake. Consider the use of an interpreter.
- Loss of trust in the doctor-patient relationship may follow. Full and frank apology may help.
- Is the patient pregnant? Review effects of clomipramine in pregnancy. If it is teratogenic you may need to consider referral for termination, and resulting emotional trauma.
- Housekeeping: Emotions may be drained, so take time before starting next consultation.

How has the incident happened?

- Has Mrs Bhatia taken clomipramine recently or in the past, remaining on the medication screen of the computer or repeat medications card if hand-held notes used?
- Has a typing or scanning error in outpatient notes been entered into the computer?
- If using a computer picking list, has the wrong drug been selected and prescribed in error by the doctor? Could it have happened with other patients?
- Has the patient presented with side-effects of the treatment?
- Has she been referred back by the hospital who may be questioning compliance?
- Have language or communication problems played a part?
- Cultural factors may contribute, eg the patient notices the error but her cultural background prevents her questioning the doctor.
- Stress may cause lack of concentration by the doctor.

Medical issues

- Need to consider potential effect of clomipramine on other medications eg FSH, side-effects, and any withdrawal effects.
- Need to inform fertility specialist. This will be professionally embarrassing and will affect future interactions with them.
- Consider need to review prescribing of unusual drugs initiated by specialists, eg interactions and side-effects.

Ethical issues

- Non-maleficence: Ensure she stops the clomipramine and check for harm as a result of treatment.
- Beneficence: Start correct medication and ensure appropriate follow-up. Is she aware of the side-effects of fertility treatment?
- Confidentiality: She may or may not wish the mistake to be discussed with family members.
- Social justice: Should fertility treatment be available in a resource-limited NHS?

Patient issues

- She may be worried about harmful effects now or in future pregnancies.
- Advise her on complaints procedure.
- Has she suffered other mistakes in the past, because of cultural or communication barriers?
- She may not trust a GP in the future.

Medico-legal issues

- Review contemporaneous notes and contact MDU.
- Inform the other partners and practice manager of what has occurred.
- If patient unhappy, encourage formal complaint to show that her concerns are properly addressed.
- Take immediate steps to prevent recurrence.

Practice issues

- Significant event audit should establish causation and prevent recurrence. Should be supportive, not punitive. Staff need to be sympathetic to Mrs Bhatia and her family. They may be keen to consult for explanations and be given an opportunity to do so. They may need to be given appointments at short notice.
- Prescribing should be reviewed, particularly if there has been an

error in a repeat prescription or as a result of a computer 'pick list'.
* Consider review of complaints procedures; are they easy for all ethnic groups to understand?
* Need for adequate medico-legal record in case of legal action.
* Support the doctor. Error has occurred. Offer time off if stressed, or time for personal development.
* Consider mentoring.
* Discuss with dispensing pharmacist. Did he notice the change in prescription? Is there any potential safety net at this level?

Answer 5

Discuss the management of the following ENT conditions, with reference to the literature:

1   Bell's palsy

This has been discussed in a review in the *British Medical Journal* in 2004[1].

Evaluation

* Most cases in adults are due to herpes zoster and herpes simplex, but need to consider alternative causes, eg Lyme's disease and serological testing should be considered in endemic areas.
* Other neurological symptoms, eg headache should prompt search for intracranial pathology.
* Thorough head and neck examination will help to exclude tumour.
* Children with Bell's palsy should be thoroughly investigated since Bell's palsy is rare and may be a sign of significant disease, eg suppurative middle-ear disease.

Short-term management

* Eye care will prevent drying and abrasion and should include lubrication and padding at night.
* High dose iv steroids given early have been shown in RCT to result in quicker resolution of symptoms and return to work, but no long-term difference in outcome.
* Combination treatment with aciclovir produces a better outcome than prednisolone alone.

Long-term management

* Psychological support, eye care and physical therapy have a place but evidence for long-term benefit is lacking

2   Benign paroxysmal positional vertigo

- This has been discussed in an editorial in the *British Medical Journal*[2]. Typically causes episodic vertigo in association with change in head position, lasting a few seconds to one minute, often provoked by such movements as turning head to one side or sitting up or lying down in bed. Need to exclude other causes, eg Meniére's disease or cerebellopontine angle tumours, usually by history.
- Diagnosed by Hallpike's manoeuvre: patient rapidly moved from sitting to lying with the head below horizontal and rotated 45° so that the affected side is lower. A positive test provokes vertigo and nystagmus with a latent period of a few seconds and lasts 30–40 seconds.
- Spontaneous remission rate high, up to 77% patients better after one month.
- Antiemetics and vestibular suppressants generally ineffective.
- Epley's manoeuvre physically moves semicircular canal debris so that it cannot cause symptoms and consists of a sequence of movements of head and trunk. A Cochrane review[3] with an odds ratio of 4.92 in favour of treatment with resolution of symptoms as an outcome.
- Where symptoms recur, patients may be taught to treat themselves. Failing this, in severe recurrent disease surgery may be used to obliterate the offending canal.

References

1   Recent developments in Bell's palsy [review]. *British Medical Journal* 2004; 329: 553–557
2   Benign paroxysmal positional vertigo [editorial]. *British Medical Journal* 2003; 326: 673
3   The Epley (canalith repositioning manoeuvre) for benign positional vertigo. *Cochrane Database of Systematic Reviews* 2002; 1.CD003162

Answer 6

Your practice is considering setting up a sleep clinic for parents of children with sleep problems. Read reference material 1.2a, an abstract from the paper entitled 'Randomised controlled trial of behavioural infant sleep intervention to improve infant sleep and maternal mood' (with copyright permission from *British Medical Journal* 324; 1062–1065).

1   Comment on the strengths and weaknesses of the methodology

Research question

- Addressed a clearly focused question, relevant to general practice.

Population

- Only looked at children aged 6–12 months. These problems are common and perhaps more significant in older children. Are the results generalisable? The control and intervention groups were broadly similar.
- Selection of participants through routine child health screening should give a good representative sample of mothers. Exclusion of those with poor English may make the study less applicable to the general population.

Intervention

- Intervention is described but impossible to say if it was standardised, eg by following a protocol.

Outcome Measures

- Outcome measures were a mixture of objective Edinburgh Postnatal Depression score, which is a validated and accepted measure, and maternal report of sleep problem (yes/no), which is subjective and open to recall bias.
- Analysis was on an intention-to-treat basis, making the results generalisable to the clinical setting.

Sources of bias

- The study was not blinded. The participants were randomised to control or intervention and masked at the analysis stage, which should reduce bias in analysis.
- The intervention was significantly different from that received by the control group. It would have been better to have given the control group three sessions of 1 to 1 consultation as well, but not given specific advice about sleep. This would have removed the possibility that it is the process of having three sessions with a friendly supportive professional that is beneficial rather than the advice about sleep.
- Inclusion criteria were maternal report of sleep problem and objective evidence of sleep problems, while at follow-up presence

of sleep problems was a subjective yes/no. Some mothers may consider it normal for children not to sleep through the night, hence answer no to the question.

Statistical methodology

- Sample size calculated to ensure power. The numbers of patients in the trial exceeded this number.
- Used regression models, a validated method of analysis.

2   **Comment on the results shown in reference material 3.2b**

Participant flow and follow-up

- Only 232 out of 738 who completed the survey were eligible to participate, and 155 agreed to do so.
- The description of the two groups lists 78 participants in each, ie 156 subjects. No mention of subjects who do not appear in follow-up, ie total of 152 participants at 2 months and 146 at 4 months.
- Were these missing people admitted to psychiatric hospital or did they commit suicide? Impossible to tell.

Significance of results

- The results show that more control mothers reported sleep problems and needed extra help at 2 months, with p values of 0.005 and 0.006, both of which are statistically significant.
- At 4 months, the differences were not significant (p = 0.26).
- The results for depressive scores only became significant after they were adjusted to account for additional professional help. This may bias the result. The results as reported were significant, with narrow confidence intervals.

Answer 7

How could you improve the care of teenagers?

Teenage healthcare is challenging: they visit surgeries infrequently, and may mistrust services. Drug misuse, psychological morbidity including depression, suicide and eating disorders are important problems, and reducing teenage pregnancy is one of the government's *Health of the Nation* targets. Factors to consider in planning teenage healthcare services include the following.

Identifying needs

- Involve teenagers in planning, eg questionnaires on needs and how to make practice appealing, or approach local school/youth groups to ask teenagers directly.
- Hold competition to design practice posters to give sense of ownership.
- Liaise with local school nurses to ascertain what services they feel are required.
- Use available evidence on strategies tried nationally to improve uptake of services.
- Audit certain areas, eg pregnancy or termination rates, parasuicide rates, to identify areas of need.

Accessibility

- Appointments to suit their needs, eg out of school hours or lunchtimes.
- Choices of personnel, eg instead of registered GP offer another GP or nurse.
- Consider offering them same day access to increase attendance.
- Be more flexible if late for appointments – inform receptionists.
- Inform patients about alternative ways to seek advice, eg telephone, email, NHS Direct.
- Consider open or walk in sessions for young people, perhaps run informally (eg by casually dressed staff) in evenings or Saturday mornings. Consider outreach health education sessions by doctors or nurses at schools or youth groups.

Promoting the practice and resources available

- Need to make teenagers feel that they are welcome and their needs are appreciated. Consider colourful, prominent posters in waiting room or on practice door stressing confidentiality and outlining services available, eg contraception, sexually transmitted diseases.
- Easily accessible leaflets on, eg eating disorders, sexual health plus prominently displayed contact numbers for services such as Family Planning clinic, GUM clinic, and teenage advice phonelines.
- Ensure all staff are welcoming to teenagers who attend – do not ask too many questions when they book appointments, etc., and respect their privacy.
- Liaise with school nurses to ensure awareness of services available. Supply free condoms.

Practice staff issues

- All staff need to be up to date on specific health needs of teenagers particularly contraception, advice on unwanted pregnancy, drug abuse. Receptionists should be aware of when to offer rapid access, eg for emergency contraception. May need training sessions. Utilise paediatric, psychiatric or fam   planning staff as resource and update regularly.
- Ensure list of local resources available for teenagers accessible to all staff.
- Help all practice staff to feel comfortable dealing with young people. Teenagers may be seen as aggressive, abusive or disrespectful but this may be a sign of fear or uncertainty. Ensure staff feel supported and safe. Consider training sessions on how to approach this age group.
- Stress importance of confidentiality.

Resource issues

- A lot can be achieved with minimal financial outlay but may entail costs in staff time; some plans (eg dedicated clinics) are expensive.
- Teenage health is a government health priority, so funds may be available. Successful pilots could be expanded to other practices.
- Diverting energies to teenage health may reduce resources available elsewhere, eg for the over 75s.

Assessing success

- Audit attendance rates and health outcomes (eg pregnancy).
- Consider patient satisfaction questionnaires to see if changes have been well received and identify areas for improvement.
- Staff meetings to discuss any problems and praise successes.

Answer 8

Mr Green and his wife come to see you for the result of his endoscopy. This showed an inoperable gastric carcinoma. How would you proceed, and what issues would you aim to cover?

Consultation considerations

Before the consultation

- Be fully informed, particularly regarding treatment options. Review latest hospital reports.

- Allow plenty of time, and avoid disturbances.

During the consultation

- Avoid euphemisms and abbreviations. Be clear and concise, short and simple.
- Find out what they know, what they fear and what they want to know.
- Encourage their thoughts and questions on the diagnosis and treatment.
- Allow plenty of time and let them dictate the pace of the consultation and have tissues ready.
- Find out how much they want their friends and families to know.

After the consultation

- Arrange to see them again when the news will have sunk in, and be available for telephone advice.
- Advise practice staff and out-of-hours providers of situation should they be called about the patient.
- Consider support services such as CancerBACUP.
- Be aware of your own emotions after the consultation.

Issues to cover with Mr and Mrs Green

Medical issues

- Be prepared for them to ask about second opinions and the possibility of alternative treatments.
- Medical needs at present? Pain? Anaemic or cachectic? Depressed?
- Be vigilant for medical and psychological complications.
- Explore their ideas, concerns and expectations regarding cancer.
- If chemotherapy is an option, explore ideas, eg about hair loss.
- When appropriate, ask Mr Green what he wants to know about the end, and how he envisages it. Is he terrified of pain, or breathing problems?
- What are his aims? One last family holiday? Encourage realism, but support these aims.

Aims of treatment

- Explain aims of treatment: Physical and psychological support, avoid suffering and preserve dignity.
- Encourage positive attitude towards palliative care, explain role of hospice and arrange for palliative care nurse to contact them if they wish.

Social issues

- Ensure social security support, eg attendance allowance. Any financial concerns?
- Assess housing needs, eg stair lift or rehousing?
- Need help with nursing?
- Encourage Mr Green to make a will, and consider an advance directive.

Psychological issues

- Prepare Mr and Mrs Green for inevitable grief reaction. Support them through this.
- Encourage openness with family members, especially estranged ones. This may prevent pathological grief later.

Other issues

- Keep an open mind about complementary therapies, eg reflexology.
- Need for hospital/hospice at-home service in the area?

Answer 9

Outline your strategies for dealing with difficult patients.

In attempting to understand difficult patients attempts have been made to categorise them, eg the dependent clinger, the entitled demander. Difficult patients are better thought of as one half of a difficult consultation and we must look to ourselves for some of the answer. Understanding the causes of 'difficult' patients helps us to deal with them.

Doctor factors

- We may promote patient anxiety or dependence by arousing unreasonable expectations, by unnecessary follow-up or through extensive investigations of minor problems.
- Our inability to identify physical symptoms of somatisation of a psychiatric illness may lead is to label these patients as 'difficult'.
- There is some evidence suggesting that overworked GPs and those who lack higher professional training and particularly training in consultation skills report more 'difficult' patients.
- Where doctors feel ill-equipped to manage a condition, eg through lack of knowledge, they may find consultations with these patients difficult.
- Patients labelled 'difficult' by colleagues may bias our approach to the consultation.

- Our failure to understand family or social dynamics may cause mutual frustration.
- Finding patients 'difficult' may represent burnout in the doctor.

Patient factors

- Complex problems often combined with difficult social circumstances may mean that patients are frustrated when we are unable to solve all their problems.
- Difficult requests or unrealistic expectations of the doctor or the health system.
- Unconventional health beliefs and non-compliance with treatment.
- Language or cultural barriers.
- Inappropriate health-seeking behaviour eg frequent attendance or unnecessary visits, a history of complaints or litigation may cause us to label them difficult.
- Patients who 'shop around' different doctors or surgeries with their symptoms are frequently seen as difficult.

Ethical issues

- Justice: We should not let prejudice influence us, but equally we are the guardians of healthcare resources. Excessive referral, investigation or treatment of demanding patients may deprive others.
- Beneficence: These patients may have genuine unidentified pathology that we should seek.
- Non-maleficence: We must protect our difficult patients from harm, eg from unnecessary treatments.
- Autonomy: we should respect patients' views about their treatment, even if different from our own.

Strategies for coping with difficult patients

For the doctor

Tailor to the different characteristics of the patient but essentially:
- Recognise your own feelings towards the patient. 'Housekeeping' before or after the consultation before you can continue with the next patient.
- Take each consultation at face value to avoid missed diagnoses.
- Recognise temptation to investigate or refer as a result of doctor anxiety or pressure.
- Sharing the problem with colleagues within the practice, mentors or in Balint groups.

- You may need to be honest and open with the patient and share feelings of frustration with them.
- Go through old notes and review diagnoses for unrecognised illness.
- Consider a contract for patients who are abusing the system or medication.
- Videotape analysis of consultations may be beneficial and highlight problem areas in communication.
- Try modifying health-seeking behaviour. Time spent in explanation or education may be beneficial in long term.
- Develop strategies for patients with lists, eg limit of two problems per consultation.
- Be aware of stress or burnout and address this.

Practice issues

- Aggressive patients require a staff policy. Staff safety is vital. Do rooms have panic alarms?
- Staff should be informed of difficult patients and discuss them.
- Practice policy for contracts or removal from list as a last resort.
- If relations have broken down, it may be in the patient's best interests to consult another doctor in the practice or consider a move to a different surgery.
- Consider significant event audit where appropriate.
- Involve the wider family or social network where appropriate.

Answer 10

Discuss the evidence relating to the following in the diagnosis and management of dementia:

1 Prevention

- The Nurses' Health Study[1] and Honolulu Heart Program[2] suggest walking may help to prevent dementia, with the most sedentary having twice the risk of the most active.
- Several studies suggest a protective effect from statins[3].
- Diet is protective, with a French study[4] showing elderly people eating fish or seafood at least once a week are at lower risk of developing dementia, including Alzheimer's disease. Folate deficiency increases the risk of Alzheimer's disease and vascular dementia and, if critically severe, can lead to a reversible dementia. Also causes depression worsening symptoms of dementia. Routine investigations should include folate and B_{12} levels[5].

2   Assessment

- The North of England Evidence Based Guidelines[6] suggest using the mini-mental test score (MMTS), as subjective complaints of memory loss are not a good indicator.
- Routine blood and urine tests should be done and Lewy body dementia should be excluded, as neuroleptics are hazardous in this group.
- Depression may be both a cause and a consequence of symptoms and should be actively sought and treated.
- In cases of sudden behavioural change other causes, eg physical or social, should be sought.
- Falls are common.
- A simple three-step assessment[7], of a single question about memory problems, assessment of global cognitive function, and neuropsychological tests found 85% of participants who had impairment at all three stages developed dementia after three years. Sensitivity was low, with over 50% of those who went on to develop dementia having no apparent initial memory problems.

3   Treatments

Gingko

- A systematic review reported in *Clinical Evidence*[8] found Gingko improved cognitive function and is well tolerated.
- *Bandolier*[9] concluded it was effective with a NNT of 7.
- Has antiplatelet effects.

Cholinesterase inhibitors

- *Clinical Evidence*[10] suggests donepezil is effective, and rivastigmine likely to be so.
- NICE guidance for these drugs and galantamine advises that they should be available on the NHS for mild to moderate Alzheimer's, should only be used for patients with a MMSE > 12/30, should only be initiated by a specialist and should only continue if MMSE > 12.
- A study in the *British Medical Journal*[11] found rivastigmine increased cognitive scores and carer-rated quality of life.
- A long term study of donepezil[12] found less evidence for benefit, since although it had a beneficial effect on MMSE scores, it did not significantly reduce admissions to care homes, care-giver time or care costs.

Atypical antipsychotics

These drugs such as risperidone are frequently used in management of agitation in dementia. A systematic review in the *British Medical Journal*[13] found limited evidence for efficacy and side-effect profile, and in 2004, the CSM advised that risperidone should not be used in elderly people due to risk of stroke.

Selegiline

- *Clinical Evidence*[10] states that there is some RCT evidence for selegiline for improving cognitive function.
- An editorial in the *British Medical Journal*[14] suggested sensory stimulation such as aromatherapy and bright light treatment was safe and effective and may have an important role in managing behavioural problems in people with dementia.

Social care

A study in the *British Medical Journal* in 2001 of care in the NHS and the private sector, found of 500 patients studied, none was receiving appropriate care and an average of 12 minutes a day was spent in constructive activities. The authors identified erroneous attitudes among staff as being partly to blame[15].

References

1 Walking and dementia in physically capable elderly men. *Journal of the American Medical Association* 2004; 292: 1447–1453
2 Physical activity, including walking, and cognitive function in older women. *Journal of the American Medical Association* 2004; 292: 1454
3 Study adds to evidence that statins reduce risk of Alzheimer's disease. *British Medical Journal* 2002; 324: 936
4 Fish, meat, and risk of dementia: cohort study. *British Medical Journal* 2002; 325; 932–933
5 Folic acid, ageing, depression, and dementia. *British Medical Journal* 2002; 324: 1512–1515
6 North of England evidence based guidelines development project: guideline for the primary care management of dementia. *British Medical Journal* 1998; 317: 802–808
7 Detection of Alzheimer's disease and dementia in the preclinical phase: population based cohort study. *British Medical Journal* 2003; 326: 245
8 Gingko biloba for cognitive impairment and dementia. Clinical Drug Invest 1999;17:301–308

9 Dementia- diagnosis and treatment. *Bandolier* 1998:48;2–3
10 Effects of treatment on cognition. *Clinical Evidence.*
11 Efficacy and safety of rivastigmine in patients with Alzheimer's disease: international randomised controlled trial. *British Medical Journal* 1999; 318: 633–640
12 Long term donepezil treatment in 565 patients with Alzheimer's disease (AD2000): randomised double blind trial. *The Lancet* 2004; 363: 9427
13 Atypical antipsychotic drugs in the treatment of behavioural and psychological symptoms of dementia: systematic review. *British Medical Journal* 2004; 329: 75
14 Sensory stimulation in dementia [editorial]. *British Medical Journal* 2002; 325: 1312–1313
15 Quality of care in private sector and NHS facilities for people with dementia: cross sectional survey. *British Medical Journal* 2001; 323: 426–427

Answer 11

Osteoporosis is a significant problem. For each of the four parts to the question, write the answers in columns under the headings 'Factors' and 'Comments and evidence':

1 Prevention of osteoporosis

- *Factor: Identifying those at risk.*
  Comment and evidence: Royal College of Physicians guidelines [1] suggest risk factors should be sought: previous fragility fracture, untreated hypogonadism, glucocorticoids >7.5 mg prednisolone a day >6 months, disease associated with risk of osteoporosis, eg hyperthyroidism, radiological osteopenia, family history and low body mass index.
  Screening vulnerable elderly people for risk factors such as gait or balance problems (eg parkinsonism), sedatives, poor vision, unsuitable accommodation may allow modification of risk factors.
- *Factor: Lifestyle measures.*
  Comments and evidence: A *British Medical Journal* review [2] suggests avoiding smoking, regular weight-bearing exercise and adequate diet are protective against osteoporosis. A meta-analysis in the *British Medical Journal* [3] suggested 1 in 8 hip fractures in women may be attributed to smoking.
- *Factor: Drugs for prevention.*
  Comments and evidence: HRT and selective estrogen receptor modulators, eg raloxifene preserve bone mass [4] and can be used in those at high risk. Raloxifene has no effect on the breast. Some

evidence that statins may reduce fracture risk[5].
Guidelines for the treatment of steroid-induced osteoporosis suggest treatment with bisphosphonates prophylactically if dose over 15 mg a day (National Osteoporosis Society).
Some evidence from observational studies that β-blockers may reduce fractures.

2 Prevention of fracture

- A systematic review confirmed benefits of exercise classes, occupational therapy input, hip protectors and medication reviews to avoid iatrogenic falls[6].
- Balance training reduces risk of falling by 30%[7].

3 Treatment of osteoporosis

- In established osteoporosis, calcium and vitamin D[8] have been shown to reduce further fractures by up to 39%, with a significant benefit being seen after 18 months[9].
- Furthermore, vitamin D seems to have an independent effect on muscle strength and decreasing falls by 50%[10].
- Bisphosphonates (Fracture Intervention Trial) have been shown to prevent vertebral and non-vertebral fractures by preventing resorption of bone[11].
- Specific estrogen receptor modulators have been shown to reduce vertebral fractures by 30% over three years[12] but no effect was seen on non-vertebral fractures. A significant decrease in numbers of new cases of breast cancer was also seen[13].
- HRT prevents fractures but needs to be taken long term. In the Women's Health Initiative among women aged 50–79 vertebral and hip fractures were reduced by 34%[14] but significant side-effects were seen.
- Salmon calcitonin prevents bone resorption and is taken nasally or by injection. This has been shown to reduce vertebral fractures by 33%[15].
- Parathyroid hormone is an anabolic hormone in bone, and injections have been shown to increase bone mass and reduce fractures by up to 90%[16].

References

1 *Osteoporosis – clinical guidelines for prevention and treatment.* London: Royal College of Physicians. 2000
2 Recent advances in rheumatology. *British Medical Journal* 2000; 321: 882–885

3 A meta analysis of cigarette smoking, bone mineral density and risk of hip fracture: recognition of a major effect. *British Medical Journal* 1997; 315: 841–846

4 Raloxifene to prevent postmenopausal osteoporosis. *Drug and Therapeutics Bulletin* 1999; 37: 33–36

5 HMG-CoA reductase inhibitors and the risk of fractures. *Journal of the American Medical Association* 2000; 283: 3205–3210

6 Preventing osteoporosis, falls and fractures amongst older people. *British Medical Journal* 1999; 318: 205–206

7 Preventing injuries in older people by preventing falls: a meta-analysis of individual-level data. *J Am Geriatr Soc* 2002; 50: 905–911

8 Effect of calcium and vitamin D supplementation on bone density in men and women of 65 years and older. *New England Journal of Medicine* 1997; 337: 670–676

9 Vitamin D3 and calcium to prevent hip fractures in the elderly women. *New England Journal of Medicine* 1992; 327: 1637–1642

10 Effect of four monthly oral vitamin D3 (cholecalciferol) supplementation on fractures and mortality in men and women living in the community: randomised double blind controlled trial. *British Medical Journal* 2003; 326: 469

11 Randomised trial of effect of alendronate on risk of fracture in women with existing vertebral fractures. Fracture Intervention Trial Research Group. *The Lancet* 1996; 348: 1535–1541

12 Reduction of vertebral fracture risk in postmenopausal women with osteoporosis treated with raloxifene: results from a 3-year randomized clinical trial. Multiple Outcomes of Raloxifene Evaluation (MORE) Investigators. *Journal of the American Medical Association* 1999; 282: 637–645

13 Continued breast cancer risk reduction in postmenopausal women treated with raloxifene: 4-year results from the MORE trial. Multiple outcomes of raloxifene evaluation. *Breast Cancer Research and Treatment* 2001; 65: 125–134

14 Risks and benefits of estrogen plus progestin in healthy postmenopausal women: principal results from the Women's Health Initiative randomized controlled trial. *Journal of the American Medical Association* 2002; 288: 321–333

15 A randomized trial of nasal spray salmon calcitonin in postmenopausal women with established osteoporosis: the prevent recurrence of osteoporotic fractures study. PROOF Study Group. *American Journal of Medicine* 2000; 109: 267–276

16 Effect of parathyroid hormone (1–34) on fractures and bone

mineral density in postmenopausal women with osteoporosis 1.
New England Journal of Medicine 2001; 344: 1434–1441

Answer 12

Read reference material 3.3a, taken from a paper entitled 'A
controlled trial of sustained-release bupropion, a nicotine
patch, or both for smoking cessation' (Reprinted with
copyright permission from *New England Journal of Medicine*
1999 340; 9: 685–692).

1   Comment on the strengths and weaknesses of the methodology

- The study addressed a clearly defined question and compared the
  three treatment options of patches, bupropion or both against
  placebo.
- Subjects were recruited by media advertisements.
  Non-English-speaking people were excluded, potentially reducing
  the generalisability of the results. Subjects were screened according
  to a set protocol, reducing inclusion bias. Allocation was
  randomised but method is unclear. Only smokers of more than 15
  cigarettes a day were included, so results may not be applicable to
  lighter smokers.
- The intervention was standardised. The study was double blinded,
  with all groups having either placebo or real patches and tablets.
  Regular biochemical monitoring of indices of smoking may have
  reinforced the intervention, making it less applicable to a primary
  care setting, but this was also true for the placebo group.
- All participants were included in analysis of outcome, ie on
  intention-to-treat, making the study more relevant to clinical care.
  The follow-up was of sufficient duration to detect real behavioural
  change.
- Outcomes were assessed as a point prevalence of not smoking at 6
  or 12 months, confirmed by objective measurement of carbon
  monoxide in expired air. This is taken to confirm continuous
  abstinence by the researchers, but could mean only recent
  abstinence. It is not clear if the participants were aware in advance
  of the date of follow-up.
- Statistical analysis is by an accepted and validated method. The
  sample size was calculated prior to the study.

2   Comment on the data in Tables 1 and 2 of reference material
3.3b

- Baseline characteristics are essentially similar, except for the
  significantly higher number of other smokers in the household for

the placebo group. They also had higher average daily consumption and expired carbon monoxide. These may make them less likely to give up.

- Subjects who were lost to follow-up or left the treatment were classified as smokers, consistent with an intention-to-treat methodology.
- Nicotine patches were not shown to be significantly effective, with odds ratios of 1.2 (0.7–1.9, $p = 0.53$) at 6 months and 1.1 (0.6–1.8, $p = 0.84$) at 12 months.
- Bupropion alone and in combination with patches was effective with odds ratios of 2.3 (1.4–3.7, $p < 0.001$) and 2.7 (1.7–4.4, $p < 0.001$) at 6 months respectively, and 2.3 (1.4–3.9, $p < 0.001$) and 3.0 (1.8–4.9, $p < 0.001$) at 12 months.
- The results suggest that nicotine patches are ineffective, although the wide confidence intervals and low p value suggest this result may be different in a larger trial population.
- The significance of the efficacy of combination therapy is unclear. If bupropion is effective on its own, then addition of anything to it would show combination therapy to be effective.

Paper 4

Answer 1

A 45-year-old businessman consults you because he has problems getting an erection. Discuss your management.

Erectile dysfunction is a common problem, affecting as many as 39% of 40-year-old men, although only a small number of them consult their GP. There are many causes, both organic and non-organic. In this consultation the GP should recognise the difficulties a man may feel when presenting with such a sensitive problem. You need to be empathic, acknowledge his concerns and reassure him about confidentiality.

History

- Take a full history. What does he mean by erectile problems? Is this new? Does he have problems initiating or sustaining erections? Early morning erections? Does he masturbate?
- Review his medical history. Does he have diabetes, vascular or neurological disease? Is he a smoker or have a heavy alcohol intake? Is he taking prescribed or illicit drugs, eg antihypertensives?
- Look for hidden agendas, eg concern about heart or neurological disease.
- Does he have signs of psychological illness, eg depression or anxiety.
- Explore psychosocial context, eg relationship problems.
- Are cultural or religious beliefs affecting his sex life?
- Why has he presented now? Is he in a new relationship? Is he worried about fertility or STDs causing his problems?
- Explore his health belief model/ideas, concerns and expectations. What does he want out of the consultation – reassurance, drugs or referral?

Examination/investigations

- Women GPs: consider chaperone/referral to male colleague for examination.
- Check BP, BMI and genitalia, looking for signs of disease including vascular disease. Check urine for glucose.

Management

- If signs of medical disorder treat accordingly, avoiding medication which will worsen problems where possible. Adjust medication if this is contributing. Advise on lifestyle modification, eg smoking.
- If psychological problems – offer to see with partner. Consider referral for psychosexual counselling. Avoid presumptions about sexuality.
- Discuss treatment options. Is he suitable for sildenafil - if he doesn't meet criteria for FP10 prescribing (eg diabetes, neurological disorders, pelvic surgery) would he pay for private prescriptions?
- Alternative treatments possible, eg Caverject. Consider referral to urologist.
- Ensure he feels supported and confirm understanding.
- Offer information about support groups.

Other issues

For the doctor

- Sensitive and potentially embarrassing topic – how comfortable do you feel in consultation? Do you yourself have sexual problems and have struggled to seek help?
- If female, would you prefer to refer him to a male colleague – patient may prefer female.
- May be unfamiliar about impotence management options – may highlight learning need.
- You may have opinions about using drugs such as sildenafil. Is it a 'lifestyle' drug or an example of government rationing?

For the practice

- Are surgery hours convenient for working patients?
- Are patients asked about reasons for consultation when booking appointments? This could deter those with sensitive problems. Advertise in reception/practice leaflet that reason does not have to be given.
- Ensure all staff are aware of confidentiality issues.
- Promotion of men's health eg specialised men's clinics. Use all opportunities for health promotion when men attend, both in consultations and with leaflets, eg about testicular self-examination, etc. Directly question men in diabetic or cardiac clinics about impotence.

For society

- Impotence is a major, largely hidden, problem causing psychological morbidity. It should be considered as important as other illnesses. Needs adequate funding.
- Why do only certain illnesses allow for NHS prescriptions whereas others are rationed?
- Limited availability of trained psychosexual counsellors.

Answer 2

'You can't teach an old dog new tricks.'

1   **How can GPs stay up to date, and what are the risks and benefits of this?**

GPs have a professional and a moral obligation to ensure they are fit to practise, and this includes a need to keep up to date. There are many ways of doing this, each with costs and benefits.

2   **Why do GPs need to keep up to date?**

- Duty of care to patients – need to be able to show that we are practising good medicine.
- Professional self-regulation relies on doctors being able to show that they are up to date.
- A GP who knows that they are up to date will have more self-confidence.
- GPs receive incentives for demonstrating that they are keeping up to date.

3   **How can GPs keep up to date and what are the risks and benefits of this?**

Attendance at educational meetings

Advantages

- Aimed at GPs, with structured format, expert speakers and relevant material. Easy to quantify time spent on educational activity.
- Educational resources (eg handouts) provided, saving time when researching information.
- Cost may be offset by drug company sponsorship.
- Sociable: Attendance offers an opportunity to meet like-minded individuals, share problems and experiences and relax away from surgery.
- Can be lunchtime or evening meetings, avoiding impact on surgery.

Disadvantages

- Often lecture-based, hence usually minimal audience participation.
- 'Experts' may not tailor content to general practice.
- Often expensive.
- Need for locums to cover duties.
- Single-handed and rural GPs may find it difficult to get locums.
- Confirmation of attendance does not confirm understanding or benefit.
- May choose subjects they enjoy, rather than areas of educational need.
- Sponsorship may introduce bias.
- Disadvantages the geographically isolated, who may not attend evening meetings.

Personal learning plans

Advantages

- Allow targeting of specific learning needs.
- Require active participation in learning.
- Encourage innovative learning, eg the internet, as well as more traditional methods.
- Less attendance at meetings; more suitable for GPs who struggle to leave the surgery.
- Encourage reflective learning.
- Cheaper than attending a series of lecture courses.
- Having a mentor is supportive for stress of general practice as well as learning.
- Encourages a rolling process of reflection and review of goals.
- Easy to do, eg with PUNS and DENS to stimulate problem-based learning.

Disadvantages

- What to put in? No universal format. May be subjective.
- May be time consuming to prepare.
- May disadvantage those with less access to information technology.
- Based on a reflective learning style. Failure to acknowledge areas of need may just result in a plan to attend lectures in a favourite area, as above.
- Goals may be set low to ensure success.
- May increase professional and social isolation.

Clinical attachments

- GPs may choose to spend a session in out-patients to improve skills in that area.

Advantages

- Experience of secondary care management of conditions.

Disadvantages

- Difficulty tailoring to specific learning needs.
- Out-patient experience may be irrelevant to primary care.
- May be seen as an extra pair of hands rather than a supernumerary.
- Attendance does not mean improvement.

Reading journals

Advantages

- Easy to do, anywhere, any time.
- Many journals are available on the internet.

Disadvantages

- Cost of journals.
- Impossible to read everything. Danger in being too selective.
- May read interesting articles, rather than those that may address a need.
- Time.

Answer 3

A 45-year-old secretary complains of intermittent loss of sensation in her left hand. You know her father has multiple sclerosis. How would you proceed?

Symptoms of sensory loss have a number of different causes including carpal tunnel syndrome, cervical spondylosis and peripheral nerve lesions.

Patient factors

- Is she aware of her father's condition?
- Likely to be anxious and worried.
- Needs to feel her concerns are taken seriously during the consultation and that she has been listened to.

- What are her ideas, concerns and expectations about her father's problems and potential diagnoses?
- Try to relate them to her psychosocial context – with respect to her job, family, hobbies, etc. What type of secretary is she? What is the impact of her symptoms on her home/working life?
- This visit may be a plea for help for her father or reflect hidden agenda, eg if sole carer not coping.

Consultation issues

- GP may be apprehensive if not confident about neurological conditions and examination.
- Patient may be well informed, which may influence the outcome or choice of management.
- Review symptoms, eg distribution of paraesthesia, any other symptoms, eg neck ache, diplopia, precipitating factors.
- Allow time to express her ideas and outline specific concerns by using open questions, reflection, etc.
- Consider psychological causes, eg anxiety and panic attacks causing paraesthesia.
- Open questions about family history give an opportunity to discuss her father.
- Do not assume concerns relate to her father's problems. She may not be associating these symptoms with his condition and may be more concerned about carpal tunnel syndrome or repetitive strain injury.
- Share findings and likely diagnoses, putting them in context of concerns and agree a management plan.

Examination/investigation

- Perform full examination relevant to differential diagnosis including CNS, CVS, fundi and neck.
- Tailor investigations to concerns: Consider ESR, glucose, TFTs, B_{12}, folate.
- If she has specific concerns about MS or suspicious findings consider a neurological opinion.

Management

- If symptoms suggestive of carpal tunnel consider simple treatment possibly with a splint or injection.
- If any other conditions identified, eg diabetes, treat accordingly.

Follow-up

- If no definitive diagnosis possible be honest, rather than bluffing.

- Arrange follow-up to allow review of progress and reporting of evolving symptoms.

Ethical considerations

- Patient autonomy: Aim for informed, shared decision making.
- Non-maleficence: Investigations may increase concern and anxiety, or have side-effects.
- Beneficence: Appropriate treatment and or referral where indicated.
- Respect confidentiality regarding both her and her father's illness when dealing with either of them.

Other issues

- Does the practice have a carers' register – if caring for her father she should be on this.
- May qualify for disability living allowance if looking after her father.
- Multiple Sclerosis Society may help with father or daughter if she has the condition.
- Any educational needs for the GP?

Answer 4

A hostel for the homeless is to be opened in your practice area. With reference to the literature, comment on the following areas of care for these patients:

1   **Barriers to care**

Patient factors

Registration

- A review in the *British Medical Journal*[1] and an editorial in the *British Journal of General Practice*[2] showed registration rate of 24% in rough sleepers. Low registration leads to poor continuity of care and preventative care.
- Study of homeless people in Leicester found 36% had experienced difficulties registering with a doctor. Most care is through accident and emergency departments[3].
- A 'cycle of reluctance'[4] has been described in which personal or reported refusal of registration further diminishes the self-esteem of the homeless person who, in expectation of refusal, does not attempt to use general practice services.

Alienation

- Hospitals and GPs are reluctant to take them on, benefits

regulations seem to penalise them, council housing departments are interested only in families and the most vulnerable, and the police may harass them.

Priorities

- Healthcare is low priority for the homeless, coming after food, shelter and money. Low rates of prescription redemption of 43% may be a reflection of this [5].

Professional factors

Attitudes

- Stereotyping: Homeless seen as alcoholics with personality disorders, who choose their lifestyle.
- Nihilism: GPs' usual interventions assume the presence of the social factors (housing, adequate nutrition and a social network) that make possible both health and treatment. May feel the absence of these will defeat any medical or psychiatric intervention.
- Organisation: Mentally ill homeless people need multi-agency help – health and social care, and housing and psychiatric care. Requires close liaison, which is the exception rather than the norm.
- GPs and many people involved in primary care lack training and experience in dealing with homelessness.
- Time: Cost disincentive for GPs under GMS.
- Philosophies of care: Some agencies operate policies that prevent or delay referral. Housing organisations assume people are always fully responsible for behaviour and may evict if a difficult patient is deemed to have made the choice.

2 Medical problems

- In a study in Birmingham, 52% of homeless children and women had experienced physical abuse [6].
- Chronic chest, skin and dental problems are frequent and may exacerbate anxiety and depression.
- Coroner's courts in London show that life expectancy was 42 years for rough sleepers [2].
- A 10-year study of the homeless in Copenhagen [7] confirmed this, finding homeless people staying in hostels, particularly young women, are more likely to die early than the general population.
- Other predictors of early death include adverse experiences in childhood, such as death of the father, and misuse of alcohol and sedatives.

3   Mental health needs

- Prevalence of schizophrenia in residents of hostels for the homeless – 9% [8].
- Homelessness may be a cause or a consequence of mental health problems.
- Homeless children are significantly more likely to have delayed development, learning difficulties and higher rates of mental health problems. These often persist after re-housing [6].
- Poor compliance with treatment and frequent drug and alcohol misuse may exacerbate problems [8].

4   Provision of care

- A study in the *British Journal of General Practice* in 2003 [9] evaluated preferences for healthcare provision of homeless in Leicester. Eighty-four per cent of homeless service users in Leicester preferred funding of 'special' health provision for homeless people.
- Such services could work in close partnership with the voluntary sector, social services and housing department [6] while contributing to education and training initiatives aimed at improving future access to mainstream services.
- An editorial in the *British Journal of General Practice* [2] stated that PMS removes time–cost disincentive through salaried posts, but there is a risk of PMS practices becoming ghettoes for the homeless, rather than integrating them in mainstream healthcare. The editorial suggested these should be a bridge, addressing immediate needs, then facilitating reintegration.
- PCTs are ideally placed for this role, and this is an ideal role for nurse practitioners.

References

1 ABC of mental health: Mental health on the margins [review]. *British Medical Journal* 1997; 315: 536–539

2 Developments in the provision of primary health care for homeless people [editorial]. *British Journal of General Practice* 2000; 52: 91–92

3 Use of hospital services by homeless families in an inner London health district. *British Medical Journal* 1989; 299: 725–727

4 *Homelessness, Health Care and Welfare Provision.* London: Routledge, 1993

5 Homeless people miss out on prescribed treatment. *British Medical Journal* 1994; 308: 135

6 Mental health problems of homeless children and families: longitudinal study. *British Medical Journal* 1998; 316: 899–902

7 10 year follow up study of mortality among users of hostels for homeless people in Copenhagen. *British Medical Journal* 2003; 327: 81

8 Comparison of prevalence of schizophrenia among residents of hostels for homeless people in 1966 and 1992. *British Medical Journal* 1994; 308: 816–819

9 How to provide for the primary health care needs of homeless people: what do homeless people in Leicester think? *British Journal of General Practice* 1999; 49: 819.

Answer 5

The senior partner in your practice has the largest prescribing bill in the health authority. What are the implications of this and how would you approach the situation?

- GPs are under increasing pressure to curb prescribing costs. There are a number of difficult issues that need to be considered in this situation.

Implications for the senior partner

Prescribing issues

- Are they frequently away (eg on PCT work), so locums are prescribing in their name?
- Are they prescribing inappropriately? Is this an indication of a wider problem?
- Are they generally a high prescriber or are certain drugs (eg PPIs) prescribed frequently?
- Is the prescribing bill high because of brand rather than generic prescribing?
- Are their patients different from those of other GPs, eg special interest in HIV with patients on expensive drugs?
- Are they an enlightened prescriber with superior knowledge of therapeutics, using drugs rather than referral for other treatment modalities, eg PPIs rather than referral for surgery in reflux?
- Are they following the NSFs to the letter?

Interpersonal issues

- How are they likely to respond to discussion of prescribing habits?
- Is there a forum where discussion of prescribing may take place in a safe environment, eg monthly prescribing meeting?
- Do they acknowledge that there is a problem?
- Why has this become an issue now? Have they upset someone in the practice or the health authority?

Implications for partners

- May be financial penalties if practice exceeds its drug budget, affecting development funds and profits.
- Clinical governance issues: If there is genuine concern about the senior partner the practice must act to prevent future charges of negligence.
- Has the situation arisen through a lack of clinical governance, eg no regular prescribing reviews?
- Discussion of these issues may provoke distrust and hostility, with implications far beyond prescribing.
- Is there a problem with repeat prescribing in general, eg failure to review medications regularly?

Implications for PHCT and practice staff

- Pharmacist: Involving a pharmacist in prescribing meetings and analysing PACT data may suggest areas for rationalisation and savings, eg changing to generics or using cheaper drugs from similar classes (eg lansoprazole rather than omeprazole).
- Practice manager: Needs to keep on top of the situation, including liaising with health authority.
- Receptionists: They are the interface between doctors and patients in any change in prescribing. They need to know how and why any changes are being made.

Wider implications

- Health authority drug overspends may require savings elsewhere, eg closure of community hospitals.
- Patients: Are patients being denied the best treatment for a condition to save money?
- GPs: Increasing use of guidelines impinges on professional autonomy. Conflict of interest between patient advocate and gatekeeper of NHS resources, increased by prescribing incentives.

Management of this situation

- Arrange a meeting with partners to discuss prescribing when all can attend.
- Ensure all stakeholders feel they have ownership of process and agree aims of prescribing review.
- Look at everyone's prescribing – what can you learn from each other?
- Agree how the prescribing review will be conducted, eg one section of the *BNF* at a time.

- Agree who will participate, eg pharmacist, one partner responsible for each section of *BNF*.
- Agree timetable for review and ensure aims auditable.
- Consider developing a practice formulary from the review.

Answer 6

A 41-year-old ex-serviceman asks for help. He complains of palpitations, nightmares and work difficulties. He smells of alcohol. His wife has seen you about relationship difficulties. Outline your approach to this problem.

This situation represents a number of challenges and potential obstacles.

Consultation style

- Requires open, unhurried style. Be aware that he may feel uncomfortable discussing personal issues.
- Respect confidentiality of all parties, especially consultations with wife about their relationship.
- Be aware of possible mental illness but also possibility of negative attitudes and stigma. Need to approach this carefully.
- Need to be aware of problems experienced by ex-servicemen.

History

- What are his principal complaints? What does he mean when he says he needs help?
- What are his ideas about his symptoms? Does he fear he has a serious heart condition?
- What are his concerns? Does he fear mental illness or Gulf War syndrome?
- What are his expectations? Referral, reassurance or a sick note?
- Review symptoms, onset and treatments taken? Is he self-medicating with alcohol or other drugs?
- Is there a clear time period of onset, eg after discharge or a traumatic incident? Ask about symptoms of PTSD.
- Any previous history of physical or mental health problems?
- Put complaints in a social context. Is he unemployed? On benefit? Has his wife threatened to leave him if he doesn't seek help?

Examination

- Aim to confirm or dispel any potential diagnoses, eg heart and blood pressure to reassure about these.

- Examine for general health. Any signs of alcoholism?
- Perform Mini-Mental State Examination, looking for signs of depression.

Investigations

- Consider ECG, 24-hour tape and blood tests to rule out organic causes.
- If concern about alcohol consumption, consider checking LFTs.

Summarise and hand-over

- Explain findings to patient and differential diagnosis.
- Offer written information on diagnoses and seek his opinions, especially if the differential diagnosis includes mental health problems.
- Offer early review by telephone or appointment to discuss concerns.
- Encourage him to bring his wife or a friend with him next time if he wishes.
- Agree a mutually acceptable approach to his problems. If appropriate suggest relationship counselling.

Management

- If PTSD likely, refer to psychiatrist.
- If depressed, consider drug treatment or referral for counselling.
- If excessive alcohol consumption, try to agree on a realistic approach to reducing this.
- Suggest Royal British Legion for advice and support.
- If taking benzodiazepines, agree on conditions for future prescriptions.
- Explain need to avoid dependence. Consider use of contract.

Other issues

- Any learning needs, eg PTSD?
- Need to be available for review and support.
- Danger of doctor dependence, if patient sees GP in a paternal role previously provided by the armed forces.

Answer 7

Your practice is considering providing a complementary medicine service to your patients. You wish to make the decision evidence based. What are the difficulties in researching complementary therapies such as acupuncture? Comment under the headings below:

1   Study design

- The gold standard is the double blind randomised controlled trial. For many complementary therapies this is not feasible. For example, in acupuncture sham treatments generate problems since they may not be a true placebo. Patients cannot be effectively blinded, since it is obvious that they are having acupuncture and not placebo. The practitioner often cannot be blinded because of the nature of complementary therapies.
- Many complementary therapies are labour intensive, which may make it very difficult to obtain data on enough patients to provide adequate statistical power.
- Objective outcomes for studies in complementary medicine are difficult to quantify, leading to reliance on subjective ones such as wellbeing, which are prone to bias.

2   Bias and confounding

- The process of treatment may be a significant confounder, eg reflexology may be very pleasurable, resulting in enhanced wellbeing separate from any supposed effect on the body's inner workings. This causes problems both in choosing objective outcome measures and in eliminating confounders.
- Studies are prone to inclusion and exclusion bias, since patients often have fixed beliefs about the relative efficacies of treatments and will select therapies they believe in (self-inclusion bias). Complementary therapists may be less likely to offer treatments to people they believe are sceptics.
- There may be problems with standardising treatments. Many complementary therapies, eg homoeopathy, are tailored to the individual and hence individual treatments cannot be compared in the way antibiotics may be compared. Another source of bias is that many complementary therapies may not have standardised training, so an acupuncturist in Croydon may be practising in a totally different way from an acupuncturist in Liverpool.
- It may be difficult for practitioners to be objective and avoid

unintentional bias, since they usually have strong faith in their own therapy.

3   Results

- There may be problems extrapolating results from individual trials to the general population. Both the therapist and the patients studied may be significantly different from the population seen in general practice.
- The data may not be amenable to standard statistical analysis, owing to heterogeneous outcomes and low sample numbers. This makes it difficult to compare both individual complementary therapies and complementary therapies and conventional medicine.
- These studies are less amenable to meta-analysis than conventional research for the same reasons: heterogeneity and lack of standardisation.
- Recent trials of homoeopathic treatments for allergy failed to show any clinical effect. Homoeopaths defended their treatments, arguing that because each individual is treated according to their unique make-up and individual problem, two individuals receiving homoeopathy for the same problem cannot be compared, let alone having two treatment arms in a large study.

Answer 8

See reference material 2.1a, taken from the paper 'A single blind trial of reflexology for irritable bowel syndrome' (with copyright permission from *British Journal of General Practice* 2002; 52: 19–23).

1   Comment on the strengths and weaknesses of the methodology

- The study aimed to answer a clearly defined question, to examine the efficacy of reflexology in the management of the core defining symptoms of IBS.
- The study was single blinded. Double blinding would not be possible since the practitioner cannot administer the treatment blind.
- The study had tight inclusion criteria: all patients were diagnosed as having IBS in accordance with the Rome criteria, a validated classification. They had all been diagnosed by a gastroenterologist, which would remove alternative diagnoses, eg Crohn's disease, which may confound.
- Patients with new symptoms, ie those who may spontaneously

improve, were excluded, as were those who had previously had reflexology, to avoid them knowing whether they were having reflexology or placebo. Including patients with chronic symptoms only potentially removes any effect of increased attention alone.
- Patient selection was via a notes search, followed by randomisation by alternation, but the numbers in each group are different: this is not accounted for in the methods and may represent bias in randomisation.
- The numbers of patients involved are small and although sample size was calculated, this was not reached, reducing the statistical power of the study.
- Control and treatment groups received identical treatments but it is not clear from the method whether they all received treatment from the same person or whether there was a standardised treatment protocol for the actual treatment rather than just a standardised process.
- Outcomes were assessed with a standardised assessment tool, reducing subjective bias in outcome reporting. Statistical assessment was by a validated method.

2   **Comment on the results in reference material 4.1b**

- 100% of randomised patients were followed up at the end of the treatment and 83% at three months.
- Baseline characteristics are given and are essentially the same.
- The fact that participants who were questioned about their treatment and who guessed did so correctly may suggest that blinding was inadequate, but 2/2 may be coincidence because the sample size was so small.
- None of the outcomes measured shows a statistically significant result, although confidence intervals and P values are not given. The range of results is wide and an effect might become apparent with larger populations.

Answer 9

Your practice is considering becoming paperless. What considerations may surround this decision?

Computers are an invaluable tool in general practice, facilitating record keeping and information flow, and we are being encouraged practically and financially to become paperless.

Benefits to practice

- Records legible and less storage space required.

- Increased data accessibility, less likely that information lost.
- Helps avoid errors – repeat prescribing, highlighting of allergies or drug interactions.
- Use for reminder systems, eg cervical smear recalls or annual blood tests.
- Templates for consultations, eg contraception or new patient checks.
- Possible direct link for IOS claims.
- Facilitates audit.
- Allows use of tools for consultation, eg decision support software for nurse-led clinics or e-mail consultations.
- Access to internet for education or patient information leaflets.
- Software for, eg anticoagulation, allows delegation of work to other staff members.
- Will facilitate flow of information between providers, eg to secondary care or out-of-hours service.

Making the decision

- Need to ensure all feel involved in planning; ownership aids acceptance.
- Ensure all staff understand benefits but listen to concerns, eg increased workload. Staff may be resistant to change, needing reassurance, adequate training, support and practical transition.
- Ensure regular meetings for problem solving.
- Have clear schedule for implementation. Will it be completely paperless, or will hospital letters/results remain as hand-held notes? Is scanning equipment required? Will a pathology link exist for results from local hospital?
- Needs clear plan – consider staggered introduction.
- Funding: Grants may be available to purchase system and training costs, but may divert resources from other services.
- Consider compatibility with PCT/hospital systems, eg pathology links.

Implementing system

- Will take time for staff to learn new skills. Cover must be arranged during this period.
- May leave practice short-staffed, resulting in increased stress, dissatisfaction or errors.
- Consider extra pay, time off in lieu or practice away-day.
- Consider training providers, eg computer company or health authority.
- Aim training at needs of different groups of staff with opportunities

to practise, ask questions and feedback.
- Consider nominated IT co-ordinator to whom problems can be referred.
- Need computers to practise on, either in practice or at outside venues.
- Consider visiting other practices with systems in place.

Potential problems

- Any system is only as good as the information put on it.
- Transferring data on to system is time-consuming – needs dedicated staff.
- Need to adhere to Data Protection Act. Enforce confidentiality issues.
- May slow down consultations initially. Patients may dislike computers.
- Sensitive information on screen visible to family members attending with patient.

Confidentiality concerns

- Temporary staff (eg temps or locum GPs) may be unfamiliar with system. Ensure clear information or training available, eg details in locum packs.
- Difficulties for branch surgeries or home visits. Will need print-outs and manual entering of details on return. Laptop computers a possibility, but expensive.
- Risk of viruses or hackers accessing confidential records – ensure adequate security system.
- If system fails, need rapid access to specialist help. Ensure practice has contingency plan.
- Will it be suitable to meet future national targets, eg electronic patient records, or need replacing in few years?

Answer 10

A 38-year-old woman with knee pain informs you during the consultation that her husband is clinical director of the local hospital. What considerations affect the consultation, and how would you proceed?

This situation requires careful consideration and delicate management.

Considerations for the doctor

- Good rapport is essential. You may expect a difficult or long consultation.

- The patient may have specific ideas, concerns and expectations, and will almost certainly have had an informal opinion from her husband before seeing you.
- You may feel a 'messenger' in the referral process but may have to accept this.
- You may well be irritated by the mention of her husband if you feel she is using this to influence you.
- Important not to assume medical knowledge and take things at her pace.
- Why has she mentioned her husband's position? This suggests you may not be her usual GP; why is she not seeing them?

Ethical considerations

- You may feel your autonomy about the management of the problem is threatened and may believe that the patient's husband will scrutinise your actions.
- You may need to reassure her regarding confidentiality.
- Can she get fair and impartial treatment at the hospital where her husband is the lead clinician?
- Social justice: Referral should be based on need. There may have to be more room for negotiation if she has fixed expectations, although her expectation may be a private referral.
- Non-maleficence: Inappropriate referral may result in unnecessary arthroscopy with possible risks.
- Beneficence: If she has a genuine problem this must be addressed.

Consultation and management

- Take full history for possible diagnostic cues.
- Any other joint problems?
- Explore psychosocial context: Does she have a job, what are her hobbies? A forthcoming special event?
- Does her husband know she has come? This should not be assumed. Has he made a tentative diagnosis or suggested to her a particular course of action?
- Summarise what worries her most and her thoughts on the likely diagnosis before examination.
- Perform an appropriate examination of the knee and other joints if required.
- Consider offering a chaperone for the examination.
- Handover: Clear explanation in appropriate language about the likely diagnosis and management options, tailored to her ideas and concerns.
- Agree a mutually acceptable management plan. Is conservative

management with analgesia appropriate? Are investigations required? Does this fit in with her expectations?
• Safety netting: Arrange follow-up.

Other issues

• If referring, it is important to include her husband's position in the letter as this may assist the next person who sees her in their consultation.
• Access: If not consulting with her regular GP, why not? Are the appointments booked? Did she feel the usual GP would be unhelpful, eg for a referral?
• Consider patient information leaflets on knee and other joint pain for simple physiotherapy or analgesia.
• Physiotherapy: Does the practice have access to physiotherapy?
• Does the practice need to look at how doctors and their families are cared for by the practice, eg confidentiality regarding notes and practice staff's access to these?
• Any learning needs?

Answer 11

With reference to current literature, discuss the following areas of primary care management of dyspepsia:

1   Investigations

• Two main clinical decisions are whether to perform endoscopy or to test for *Helicobacter pylori*.
• NHS guidelines for 2-week suspected cancer referrals – urgent upper gastrointestinal endoscopy indicated for following alarm symptoms:
  – dysphagia
  – dyspepsia at any age with weight loss, anaemia or vomiting
  – dyspepsia with risk factors, eg Barrett's oesophagus, family history
  – jaundice or upper abdominal mass.
• NICE guidelines[1] suggest routine endoscopy is unnecessary in a patient of any age without alarm symptoms, but in the over 55-year-old age group, endoscopy may be used if:
  – empirical treatment with a PPI or test and treat are unsuccessful
  – when patients have ongoing needs for NSAIDs
  – previous ulcer
  – anxiety about cancer.
• For most, initial decision is empirical PPI or test and treat;

insufficient evidence about which is better.

- Test and treat may be a C13 breath test, stool antigen or serology. Positive patients should receive seven days of a PPI and either metronidazole and clarithromycin 250 mg (PMC250) or an amoxicillin and clarithromycin 500 mg (PAC500) regimen. Re-testing is not usually indicated, however, treatment failures are common due to rapid develo ...ent of resistance; persistent symptoms may require re-testing or re-treating [2]. In an RCT, test and treat was acceptable to patients, reassuring and economically superior [3].
- It does not make reflux better. Eradication rates are higher in those who drink alcohol, compared with those on the same regimen who do not [4].

2 Interventions

- All patients should have medication reviewed for causative drugs, eg bisphosphonates.
- Advice on smoking, weight reduction, healthy eating, avoiding precipitants such as alcohol.
- Patients should be reviewed regularly and have medication stepped down or stopped where possible.

The NICE guidelines [1] suggest the following interventions.

Interventions for GORD

- Full dose PPI for one to two months then step down to the lowest dose that controls symptoms.

Interventions for peptic ulcer disease

- *H. pylori* eradication in *H. pylori* positive patients with ulcers.
- Patients on NSAIDs – stop these where possible.
- Offer full dose PPI or H_2RA for two months and treat for *H. pylori* if present [1,2,5].

Interventions for non-ulcer dyspepsia

- Endoscopically proved non-ulcer dyspepsia should be treated for *H. pylori* if present, followed by symptomatic treatment [5].
- Estimated that if NICE guidelines were universally applied this would save £40–£50 million per annum. A study of patients and GPs' attitudes towards PPIs in the *British Journal of General Practice* in 2001 suggested that the notions of profligate prescribers and lifestyle drugs are wrong, the majority of patients being elderly with complex health needs [6].

- NICE guidelines also suggest encouraging patients to use treatment prn.

Surgery

- In severe GORD if PPI ineffective, surgery may be indicated, however there is some debate about the merits of laparoscopic rather than open fundoplication [7].

References

1 Dyspepsia – management of dyspepsia in adults in primary care. NICE Clinical Guideline 17. August 2004. www.nice.org.uk
2 ABC of the upper gastrointestinal tract. Management of *Helicobacter pylori* infection. *British Medical Journal* 2001; 323: 1047–1050
3 Randomised trial of endoscopy with testing for *Helicobacter pylori* compared with non-invasive *H pylori* testing alone in the management of dyspepsia. *British Medical Journal* 2002; 324: 999
4 'Relation between alcohol consumption and the success of Helicobacter pylori eradication therapy using omeprazole, clarithromycin and amoxicillin for 1 week' *European Journal of Gastroenterology and Hepatology* 2002; 14: 291–296
5 Role of Helicobacter pylori infection and non-steroidal anti-inflammatory drugs in peptic ulcer disease: a meta analysis. *The Lancet* 2002; 359: 14–22
6 Proton pump inhibitors: perspectives of patients and their GPs. *British Journal of General Practice* 2001; 51: 703–711
7 Laparoscopic or conventional Nissen fundoplication for gastro-oesophageal reflux disease: randomised clinical trial. *The Lancet* 2000; 355: 170–174

Answer 12

'Statins: a panacea for all ills?'

Comment on this statement, with reference to current evidence.

Statins have been shown to be beneficial in many systems of the body. Their effectiveness can be discussed under several heads:

Cardiac effects

- A paper in the *British Medical Journal* in 2003 [1] suggested giving a poly pill containing a statin, folic acid, aspirin, a thiazide, β-blocker

and ACE inhibitor to everyone over the age of 55 and everyone with
established ischaemic heart disease.
- This approach was based on meta-analyses of individual studies
  and suggested a possible reduction of 88% for cardiac events and
  80% for stroke, with 8–15% drop-out rate due to side-effects.

Primary prevention of ischaemic heart disease

- A meta-analysis in the *British Medical Journal* in 2000[5] showed a
  reduction of 30% in cardiac events.
- WOSCOPS showed benefit of treating asymptomatic men with high
  cholesterol levels[3], while AFCAPS/TexCAPS showed benefits of
  treating asymptomatic men and women with normal cholesterol[4].

Secondary prevention of ischaemic heart disease

- 4S study showed a relative risk reduction of 30% in statin users with
  previously high cholesterol[5].
- CARE study showed benefits in secondary prevention for people
  with normal cholesterol[6].
- Heart Protection Study[7] suggests that five years of statin treatment
  typically prevents heart attacks, strokes or other major vascular
  events in:
  - 1 in 10 people who have had a heart attack
  - 8 in 100 people with angina or some other signs of coronary
    heart disease
  - 7 in 100 people who have ever had a stroke
  - 7 in 100 people with diabetes.

Effects on bone

- Evidence from the UK General Practice Research Database suggests
  statins lower fracture rates[8].

Effects on CNS

Depression

- Long-term use of statins reduced levels of depression by 30–40% in
  an observational study. This was independent of cholesterol
  reduction but differed between statins with different levels of
  lipophilicity, suggesting a CNS effect[9].

Stroke

- Systematic review supports use of statins in people with prior stroke, coronary heart disease, and a cholesterol concentration greater than 5 mmol/l (or LDL cholesterol concentration > 3 mmol/l) [10].

Alzheimer's disease

- A study in the *British Medical Journal* in 2002 [11] provided evidence that statins are associated with a 79% reduction in the risk of developing Alzheimer's disease.

Macular degeneration

- A cross-sectional study in the *British Medical Journal* in 2001 [12] suggests patients on statins have significantly lower rates of macular degeneration.

Other effects

- There is some evidence that statins may be useful in preventing transplant rejection [13].

Problems with statin use

- Numerous studies suggest that many people fail to get the full benefit either due to lack of access (ie not offered statins) [14] or due to intolerable side-effects, with discontinuation rates up to 30% in one study [15].

References

1 A strategy to reduce cardiovascular disease by more than 80%. *British Medical Journal* 2003; 326: 1419
2 Use of lipid lowering drugs for primary prevention of coronary heart disease: meta-analysis of randomised trials. *British Medical Journal* 2000; 321: 983
3 Prevention of coronary heart disease with pravastatin in men with hypercholesterolemia. *New England Journal of Medicine* 1995; 333: 1301–1307
4 Primary prevention of acute coronary events with lovastatin in men and women with average cholesterol levels. Results of AFCAPS/TexCAPS. *Journal of the American Medical Association* 1998; 279: 1615–1622
5 Scandinavian Simvastatin Survival Study Group. Randomised trial of cholesterol lowering in 4444 patients with coronary heart disease: the Scandinavian Simvastatin Survival Study (4S). *The Lancet* 1994; 344: 1383–1389
6 The effect of pravastatin on coronary events after myocardial

infarction in patients with average cholesterol levels. *New England Journal of Medicine* 1996; 335: 1001–1009

7 Statins are the new aspirin. *British Medical Journal* 2001; 323: 1145

8 HMG-CoA reductase inhibitors and the risk of fractures. *Journal of the American Medical Association* 2000; 283: 3205–3010

9 'Long-term statin use and psychological well-being,' *Journal of the American College of Cardiology* 2003; 42: 690–696[Q20]

10 Cholesterol lowering with statin drugs, risk of stroke, and total mortality. An overview of randomized trials. *Journal of the American Medical Association* 1997; 278: 313–321

11 Study adds to evidence that statins reduce risk of Alzheimer's disease. *British Medical Journal* 2002; 324: 936

12 Risk of macular degeneration in users of statins: cross sectional study. *British Medical Journal* 2001; 323: 375–376

13 'Statins as a newly recognised type of immunomodulator,' *Nature Medicine* 2000; 6: 1399–1402

14 Statins: underused by those who would benefit [editorial]. *British Medical Journal* 2000; 321: 971–972

15 'Discontinuation rates for use of statins are high,' *British Medical Journal* 2000; 321: 1084

Paper 5

Answer 1

See reference material 3.1a, an extract from 'Survival outcome of care by specialist surgeons in breast cancer: a study of 3786 patients in the west of Scotland' (with copyright permission from *British Medical Journal* 1996; 312: 145–148).

1   Comment on the design of the study

- The study is a retrospective cohort study, and includes all the patients treated in the west of Scotland over the study period. This form of study is appropriate for comparing outcome between two groups. These were identified from the cancer registry and confirmed histologically, which should give universal coverage with minimal selection bias.
- Classification of surgeons as specialists by one person on the basis of local perception is extremely subjective and introduces a powerful source of bias.
- Follow-up was at least five years from diagnosis, making the results comparable with the standard index of mortality, the 5-year survival rate.
- The analysis of the data took account of other potential confounders such as tumour size, age, socio-economic status and nodal involvement. It did not take into account co-morbidity, which may be a confounder.
- The outcome measures included 10-year mortality, but follow-up only continued up to 1993, five years after the last cohort was recruited. This may allow reporting bias to influence results, with patients dying after the end of the study but within 10 years of diagnosis not being included.

2   Comment on the results in table 1 (reference material 5.1b)

- The results suggest that there is a statistically significant difference in survival between specialist surgeons and non-specialist surgeons.
- This difference persists when age, deprivation, nodes and tumour size are accounted for.

- The confidence intervals for all of these favour the results, suggesting they are true.

3   Give possible alternative explanations

- Specialist surgeons may provide better treatment and may refer more appropriately for adjuvant treatment, resulting in better survival rates.
- The study does not account for tumour type, eg ductal carcinoma in situ vs fungating tumour, which may affect the results.
- Similarly, no account is made of the use of adjuvant treatment, eg tamoxifen, chemotherapy or radiotherapy, which are more likely to be available in large specialist hospitals.
- Non-specialists are more likely to work in hospitals with small patient numbers and it has been shown that patient volume affects outcomes.
- The west of Scotland is a diverse area with many remote communities distant from the centres of excellence. Patients with advanced disease or other medical problems may not be referred or may decline referral to these centres on grounds of distance or transport difficulties. These may not be detected by deprivation scores.
- The use of lymph node involvement in the analysis relies on lymph nodes being sampled. This is more likely to be done by specialist surgeons.

Answer 2

A concerned father brings his 14-year-old son asking you to screen him for drugs. Discuss the issues this raises.

Drug misuse is an increasing problem among teenagers that has not only risks for health but also implications for education, family relationships and crime.

Doctor issues

- Responsibility to father and son. Need good rapport and address needs of both.
- Be non-judgemental/advocate for both. Assure confidentiality.
- Possibly long, difficult consultation. Best to see both father and son individually and together. Both may be angry; try to defuse tension.
- Be aware of your own feelings. Consider debriefing with colleagues over a cup of tea afterwards.

- May identify lack of knowledge on issues of consent, drug misuse or efficacy of testing.
- May feel out of depth and prefer to refer to local drugs service/paediatrician.
- Consider asking medical defence society for advice.

Patient issues

For the father

- Why attend today? Is son in trouble with police or school, or is he unwell?
- What are his ideas about drug use? Does he or other family member use drugs?
- What does he know about drug screening? Needs to understand implications for son, ie illegal activity may affect employment prospects.
- Need to inform him about issues of consent, ie son's autonomy and right to refuse testing under Children Act. Parents do not have automatic right to override.

For the son

- Need to assess competence – can refuse to consent if understands purpose of procedure and the consequences of the results.
- If using, may not see as a problem especially if 'soft' drugs, eg cannabis. May need education.
- Assess knowledge of risks of drug misuse, eg HIV/hepatitis if injecting. Consider examination. Opportunity for health promotion.
- Assess for psychological problems (eg depression) and problems at home or school (eg bullying or abuse).
- May resent father's interference – try to help him understand father's concerns.
- May be pleased at opportunity to seek help, eg may not have had the courage to admit it previously.
- Advise about availability for help, eg local drugs service, helplines, teenage psychiatric services.

Practice issues

- Is surgery adolescent friendly? Are there leaflets/posters on related topics and where to seek help?
- Are all staff (eg nurses) aware of issues of confidentiality and consent? Are staff up to date on signs of drug abuse and local management options?

- Drug abusers can be aggressive – are safety procedures in place?
- Does practice have treatment policy? One GP seeing all drug abusers or refer all to drugs service?

Local issues

- What services are available in the area to help drug abusers? Adequate provision and funding?
- Education may need outreach by drug workers to schools/youth groups.
- Involve local media in campaigns on risks and where to seek help.

National/society issues

- Need to address situations that cause drug abuse – deprivation, lack of activities for youngsters.
- Media portrayal of drug use may glamorise it.
- Experimentation is part of adolescence so need adequate education for both children and parents of the risks.
- Should responsibility for preventing drug abuse rest on the NHS rather than parents and schools?
- As a society do we need open debate or more liberal policies on 'soft' drugs, as in the Netherlands?
- Drug treatment services and advertising campaigns need more resources.
- Need to tackle drug smuggling and dealing to reduce availability on streets.

Answer 3

A 33-year-old man asks to be referred for a circumcision, informing you that this was suggested after a consultation over the internet for premature ejaculation. Outline your management of this consultation.

Sexual problems are common, often involving an underlying psychological or psychosexual reason. This patient has taken time to seek solutions to his problem on the internet, showing his concern about his symptoms. The consultation may be difficult for both doctor and patient.

Approach to consultation

- Develop rapport by listening to the patient's request, encouraging him through open questions. Acknowledge his possible embarrassment, and the importance of the problem to him.

- GP may feel embarrassed, irritated or threatened by patient seeking advice from the internet.
- Are you comfortable with taking a sexual history and the treatment options?
- Avoid presumptions about sexuality.
- Take a full sexual history: avoid jargon and use the patient's own terms.
- What does he mean by premature ejaculation? How long has the problem been going on?
- Explore psychosexual situation: Any underlying psychological difficulties? New partner? Is the relationship threatened by the problem? Any other stressors at home or at work?
- Has he already tried other methods of treatment?
- Explore ideas, concerns and expectations: Any other reason for his request, eg does his partner wish him to be circumcised? Are there religious reasons?
- Offer to read the internet information.
- Be honest if you are unfamiliar with circumcision as a treatment for premature ejaculation.
- As patient's advocate, explain need to assess the information for bias, poor research or potential risks.
- Examination: If indicated from history, offer a chaperone if needed.
- Summarise his concerns and expectations. Agree a management plan with him putting this in the context of the request.
- Offering a joint consultation with his partner may be helpful and might identify psychosexual problems. Are they concerned about the premature ejaculation?
- Discuss other treatment options which include stop/start technique, books such as *Treat Yourself To Sex*.
- If necessary consider referral for psychosexual therapy (eg to Relate), family planning or a private counsellor rather than a referral to a urologist.

Ethical issues

- Non-maleficence: Avoid harm by what may be an inappropriate referral for an operation. Explain the potential for bogus advice on the internet. Explain possible detrimental health effects.
- Beneficence: Avoid belittling the patient's request and involve him in the management plan.
- Autonomy: For the patient – respect his request and acknowledge his efforts in seeking a solution to his problem; for the doctor – ability to decide on treatment or management plan.
- Confidentiality: Explain you will not discuss the problem with his partner without his consent.

Wider issues

- Internet information
  - Pros: Potential for increased availability of information. Many sites, eg those of patient support groups, the Royal Colleges or charities, are good quality, allowing patients to learn about their diagnosis and be well informed in consultations.
  - Cons: Unfiltered information may be biased, poorly researched or suggest treatments which can be purchased directly, bypassing usual doctor.
  - Medicolegal considerations: Questions over where responsibility lies for internet consultations that may be in other countries.
- Any learning needs?
  - Well-man clinics may allow opportunity to discuss sexual health issues with the doctor or practice nurse in a more informal clinic setting.
  - Are there any patient information leaflets on sexual problems which could be made available within the practice?

Answer 4

Patients with cardiological conditions are increasingly being cared for in primary care. Discuss the latest developments with regard to the following areas:

1 **Atrial fibrillation**

Rate or rhythm?

- Data from trials of DC cardioversion (AFFIRM study)[1] and chemical cardioversion[2] show no benefit for mortality, quality of life or risk of stroke.

Pacemakers?

- Dual chamber pacing for paroxysmal atrial fibrillation may reduce incidence and progression to chronic atrial fibrillation, but no benefits are seen for two years[3].

Antiplatelet or anticoagulant?

- A paper in 2003 in the *Archives of Internal Medicine*[4] suggested to carry out risk stratification before decide to guide decision making.
- Irrespective of age, for patients with no additional risk factors (no past medical history, cardiovascular examination/TIA, no IHD, BP or diabetes) risks of warfarin > benefits.

- There are no data as yet on clopidogrel vs aspirin, so aspirin should be considered first choice as an antiplatelet, unless contraindicated.
- Ximelagatran, a direct thrombin inhibitor has been shown in direct comparisons with warfarin to be as effective in preventing stroke, with a better side-effect profile and similar rates of major bleeding but less minor bleeding. More importantly, it does not require regular monitoring (SPORTIFF III trial [5]).

2   Cardiac rehabilitation

- A Cochrane review in 2004 [6] showed a 31% reduction in mortality in cardiac rehabilitation patients.
- The SIGN guidelines [7] suggest four phases of cardiac rehabilitation:
  – full evaluation and education in hospital
  – psychological and emotional support in the early discharge period
  – primary healthcare team then takes over to provide structured exercise training and psychological support
  – long-term maintenance of physical activity and lifestyle change.
- Patients with co-morbidities, eg diabetes, require particular attention since they tend to have greater adverse risk factors such as high BMI, hypertension and adverse lipids [8].

3   Antiplatelet therapy for ischaemic heart disease

- Up to 45% of the population is resistant to aspirin, and clopidogrel is an effective alternative for secondary prevention and in acute non-ST myocardial infarction (CAPRIE [9] and CURE [10] trials).
- Following angioplasty dual platelet blockade for one year rather than one month produces fewer ischaemic events [11].

References

1 Atrial fibrillation follow up investigation of rhythm management (AFFIRM). A comparison of rate control and rhythm control in patients with atrial fibrillation. *New England Journal of Medicine* 2002; 347: 1825–1833

2 Management of atrial fibrillation – radical reform or modest modification? *New England Journal of Medicine* 2002; 347: 1883–1884

3 Implantable devices for the treatment of atrial fibrillation. *New England Journal of Medicine* 2002; 346: 2062–2068

4 A clinical prediction rule to identify patients with atrial fibrillation and a low risk for stroke while taking aspirin. *Archives of Internal Medicine* 2003; 163: 936–943

5 Stroke prevention with the oral direct thrombin inhibitor ximelagatran compared with warfarin in patients with non-valvular atrial fibrillation (SPORTIF III): a randomised controlled trial. *The Lancet* 2002; 362: 1691–1698

6 Exercise-based rehabilitation for coronary heart disease (Cochrane review). In: the Cochrane Collaboration. *Cochrane Library*. Issue 3.

7 www.sign.ac.uk

8 Results of cardiac rehabilitation in patients with diabetes mellitus. *Journal of the American College of Cardiology* 2004; 93: 81–84

9 A randomised, blinded, trial of clopidogrel versus aspirin in patients at risk of ischaemic events (CAPRIE). *The Lancet* 1996; 348: 1329–1339

10 Clopidogrel in unstable angina to prevent recurrent events trial investigators. Effects of clopidogrel in addition to aspirin in patients with acute coronary syndromes without ST elevation. *New England Journal of Medicine* 2001; 345: 494–502

11 Early and sustained dual oral antiplatelet therapy following percutaneous coronary intervention: randomised controlled trial. *Journal of the American Medical Association* 2002; 288: 2411–2420

Answer 5

A 15-year-old girl complains of problems 'down below'. What issues surround this consultation?

This embarrassing problem has a number of causes and is a potentially difficult consultation. Good rapport and sensitivity are vital.

Factors to consider

- For a male doctor: Is she happy to see you? May want to see a female GP or nurse.
- May need female chaperone, especially for examination.
- She is a minor. Do you feel happy to see her alone? Are parents aware she is attending?
- Need to ensure she is competent to consent to questioning or examination. If concerns about possible abuse, consider advice from paediatricians.
- Assure of confidentiality unless suspected abuse or rape. Her safety is paramount and you may be obliged to notify social services or police in this situation.
- Do you feel comfortable discussing sex with a 15-year-old girl? You

may be embarrassed, or have strong views on under-age sex, especially if you have teenage daughters. Do not allow feelings to affect consultation.
• What is your knowledge of vaginal discharge; if not confident, consider family planning/GUM clinic referral. May highlight learning need.

History

• Establish her concerns. Is she worried about STDs, pregnancy, gynaecological disease, eg cancer or infertility? Has a friend or family member recently developed any of these?
• How long has discharge been present? Discuss nature of discharge, any bleeding, abdominal pain or itch? Has she had it before? Recent antibiotics or steroids causing candidiasis?
• Is she sexually active? Contraception or condoms? LMP, establish risk of pregnancy.
• Does a partner have symptoms?
• Is her agenda contraceptive advice or seeking advice about STDs? Is she 'Gillick' competent?
• Consider if she could be in a non-consensual sexual relationship – rape or abuse. If partner is older, having sex with a minor is illegal even if she consents.
• Does she have psychological illness, eg depression, causing preoccupation with health?

Examination

• Consider vulval/speculum examination to take HVS/chlamydial swabs and look for signs of abuse.
• Consider pregnancy test.
• General examination, eg for signs of diabetes, eczema.

Management

• Offer treatment depending on likely cause.
• Consider stat treatments for increased compliance, eg azithromycin.
• Discuss sexual health. Provide details of GUM/family planning clinic for further advice. Give leaflets.
• Discuss contraception and encourage to return.

Issues for practice

• How teenage friendly is the practice? Need easy access to appointments with choice of medical staff, posters and leaflets

about sexual health, contraception. Emphasise confidentiality.
- Need easy access to chaperones for male GPs.
- Consider outreach to schools or youth groups to educate about services available and sexual health.
- Co-ordinate efforts with school nurses.

Local issues

- Teenagers important target group for funding.
- May need to improve access to services, eg teenage walk-in clinics outside school hours.
- Use local media to highlight issues on sexual health and how to seek help.

National issues

- Health of nation/sexual health and HIV policies target sexual health and teenage pregnancy rates.
- Ensure adequate sex education in schools.
- Try to remove some of the taboos on discussing sex openly in society.
- National campaigns, eg to screen for *Chlamydia*, advocate safe sex, etc.
- Funding for sexual health advice and contraception, eg more family planning and GUM clinics.

Answer 6

A 48-year-old woman asks for a repeat thyroxine script, started recently for weight loss by one of your partners. Her BMI is 26 and no thyroid blood tests are recorded. How do you manage this request?

This request puts the doctor in an awkward position, as there appears to be no clear clinical indication for the prescription. It raises a number of issues.

Ethical considerations

- Autonomy: We reserve the right to act according to our principles, including not to prescribe.
- Non-maleficence: Do not cause harm by unsafe prescribing.
- Beneficence: Not prescribing avoids risk to physical health but harm may arise from loss of trust in her doctor or from feeling a treatment is being withheld.

Consultation considerations

- Need for tact and a non-confrontational style. Patient expecting a repeat script may be alarmed if questioned in detail.
- Establish the facts: Is this a safe prescription request?
- Who commenced the treatment? Care needed to avoid loss of trust in the doctor-patient relationship.
- Why was the prescription started?
- Have any tests been done that are not recorded in the notes?
- What does she understand about her treatment and the reasons for commencing thyroxine?
- Was script requested by the patient, eg after hearing of people losing weight this way?
- Review previous attempts at weight loss, eg diet/exercise/weight watchers.
- Explore her health beliefs regarding weight loss.
- Any cautions or contraindications for thyroxine use, eg ischaemic heart disease.
- Any side-effects of treatment, eg angina, palpitations or dyspnoea.
- Examine patient to check for signs of hypothyroidism or hyperthyroidism.

Management options

Immediate

- If unable to prescribe, explain why but respect her relationship with her usual GP. Explain that different doctors often manage clinical situations in different ways.
- Suggest she see your partner to discuss the prescription.
- Review notes looking for diagnosis of hypothyroidism or thyroxine treatment.
- Suggest alternative weight loss management, eg practice nurse clinic.
- Risks to doctor-patient relationship of refusal may warrant a limited script after explaining risks.
- Importance of good records.

Future

- Discuss with the GP in a non-confrontational way, eg 'I noticed Mrs . . . was on thyroxine but I wasn't quite sure why . . . ', allowing her GP to explain the prescription.
- Was this on specialist advice and has there been inadequate documentation?

- Has the doctor recently read an article that suggested the treatment?
- Has the doctor felt pressurised to prescribe to end a difficult consultation or to please the patient?
- Discuss at practice prescribing or significant event meeting.
- If the partner is unrepentant, you may need to contact LMC/GMC. You have a duty to act if colleagues are unsafe.

Practice issues

- Potential conflict between the partners; handle with care. Avoid jumping to conclusions.
- Clinical governance. Audit of other patients on thyroxine and weight loss management. Is this a one-off, or one of many?
- Is it a problem of inadequate record keeping or aberrant prescribing?
- Does it identify learning needs for the doctor involved?
- Anticipate the possibility of a complaint.

Wider issues

- No national guidelines on obesity management support the routine use of thyroxine. Specialist clinics may prescribe thyroxine under close supervision, and this difference in medical practice and opinion can lead to conflicts.
- Medico-legal aspects: Risk of serious side-effects eg AF or chest pain occur on inappropriately prescribed treatment. Contact medical defence organisation.
- Local PCO/CHImp may become involved if found to be a widespread prescribing issue.

Answer 7

What are the difficulties in dealing with doctors as patients?

Ethical issues

- Confidentiality: Remain professional and keep consultations within the surgery. Avoid the temptation of continuing consultations in a social setting.
- Justice/equality: Should treat as any other patient.
- Autonomy: Doctor may feel under pressure to pursue clinical course at variance with own diagnosis. Need to acknowledge patient's ideas and expectations about a particular course of action.

Consultation issues

- Doctor's feelings: May find it a difficult consultation. May feel under scrutiny or apprehension/ego boost that colleague is coming to consult.
- Time-keeping: May be stressed or embarrassed if running late. Effect on previous/subsequent patients if try to catch up prior to the consult or if over-run.
- Aim for patient-centred approach, get to the bottom of concerns and expectations.
- Need to share clinical findings and clinical diagnosis, and agree management plan.
- Professional status, eg seniority. The patient may be more knowledgeable about or more experienced in the problem presented. Should they be referred to another partner or specialist?

Patient issues

- Often unregistered, and consulting GP may not have their old medical records.
- May expect to be treated differently, eg invited into the reception office rather than waiting in the waiting room.
- Frequently self-medicate before consultation, clouding the clinical picture or delaying diagnosis.
- They may also be treating other family members or attending out of courtesy but expecting a referral to a specialist.
- Psychological/relationship/drug/alcohol issues. High incidence of all these in the medical profession. Embarrassment may prevent attendance.
- Patient's feelings: May have inaccurate health beliefs, eg a consultant psychiatrist thinking he has bowel cancer when he has piles, and have unrealistic expectations of treatment/referral.

Practice issues

- Should GPs working in a practice register with another practice to avoid conflicts of interest?
- Preferential treatment, eg may expect to be put straight through to GP to discuss case/investigations, or to be given contact number for out of hours.
- Costs: More likely to request expensive medication or investigations (which may be unnecessary).
- Higher referral rate to outpatients for second opinions or treatment.
- Is there a policy relating to notes for staff/professional colleagues? Notes need to be secure, eg by blocking access via security levels on computers or locking hand-held notes in a separate area.

Answer 8

You are a member of a working party carrying out a review of community care of patients with Parkinson's disease. You are keen to make any decisions evidence based.

1 Outline how you would gather your evidence

- The evidence should be gathered by first deciding on a research question, eg 'Are community nurses effective in preventing hospital admissions in Parkinson's disease?'
- The next stage is to agree a search strategy, eg all medical and nursing journals published in English.
- Searches are made of databases (eg Medline, Cochrane Collaboration) and local resources (eg medical library).
- Supplementary information can be gained from asking interested parties, eg local neurologist.
- Once the search is complete, the results should be screened. The screening process should be agreed by stakeholders to avoid bias and should be hierarchical, eg first preference for systematic reviews, then randomised controlled trials, and then down to case reports.
- The screening should also take into account relevance of location, eg UK studies more relevant to UK practice, quality of journal (Is it peer reviewed?) and quality of research.

2 Details of the methodology of one paper being discussed ('Effects of community based nurses specialising in Parkinson's disease on health outcomes and costs: randomised controlled trial', *British Medical Journal* 2002; 324: 1072–1075) are given in reference material 5.2a. (With copyright permission from the *British Medical Journal*.) Comment on the strengths and weaknesses of the study design, intervention and sampling methods

Strengths

- Set in UK primary care, with practices selected at random in nine health authority areas each also selected at random from all over England, making the data more likely to be applicable in general.
- All practices in the selected areas were invited to participate, reducing risks of inclusion bias. Exclusion criteria were minimal, which improves generalisability.
- The length of the study and the number of participants were sufficient to detect any genuine effects, and a sample size was calculated to ensure power.

- Nurses received standardised training and resource package and had standardised responsibilities.
- Assessment of outcomes was by trained lay interviewers with standardised tools. This would reduce bias.
- Outcome measures were clear and objective.

Weaknesses

- It is unclear whether the study was limited to Parkinson's disease or all patients with parkinsonism.
- It is not possible to tell where the areas studied are. They may be scattered all over the UK, giving a heterogeneous population representative of the country, or they may be clustered in a small area.
- The control group received no extra help of any description. It may be that the process of someone visiting is beneficial, rather than any specific nursing intervention, and this may bias the quality of life assessment.
- The nursing time use study was only done over two 1-week periods.
- These periods may not be representative of the 2-year period and the nurse may alter their working pattern in the knowledge that they are being observed.
- The intervention is difficult to quantify through time use study. There is no objective recording of what the nurses were actually doing, eg telephone calls could be to arrange physiotherapy or could be to cancel the newspapers for a patient.

Answer 9

Extracts from the results of the paper entitled 'Effects of community based nurses specialising in Parkinson's disease on health outcomes and costs: randomised controlled trial' (*British Medical Journal* 2002; 324: 1072–1075) are given in reference material 5.3a. (With copyright permission from *British Medical Journal*.)

1   How do the results support a decision in favour of the intervention?

- The subjective change in general health between the groups was significantly better in the intervention group.

2   How do the presented results support a decision against the intervention?

- There was no significant difference between the intervention and control groups in severity of disease, mortality or fractures.

- No differences were observed in the objective measures of wellbeing.
- The only statistically significant improvement was not a primary outcome and it is unclear when this was included. This may be a source of bias.

3 **Comment on the analysis of the costs**

- Cost analysis shows that the intervention group were more expensive than the control group, but this includes the cost of the nurses. When this is allowed for, the costs are almost equal. A breakdown of the costs shows that institutional costs, primary care and drug costs were lower for the intervention group. These results suggest that although the overall costs may be the same, the money may be being spent differently, eg increased home help costs allowing patients to stay at home rather than going into institutions.

4 **Are there any other explanations for the lack of effect in the results?**

- The nurses were newly trained. They may have been on a steep learning curve, spending much of their time learning local systems and increasing their expertise.
- The nurses spent much of their time in administrative tasks and driving. It may be that if they concentrated more on clinical interventions they would have been more effective.
- No standardised diagnosis of Parkinson's disease. Relying on GP records may bring in patients with other conditions misdiagnosed as Parkinson's, eg essential tremor, although if these were evenly distributed between control and intervention groups this would have had less impact.

Answer 10

You see a 55-year-old woman who works in a pottery with her husband. She tells you she has been seen at the walk-in centre, where she was told that she should be referred to the allergy clinic regarding a rash. What issues does this raise, and how would you proceed?

This problem raises several difficult issues and requires a considered approach to produce a mutually acceptable result.

Consultation issues

- Preconceived agenda: Need to acknowledge concerns and expectations and be open to negotiation.

- Take account of her husband. He may require a different style of consultation.
- Difficult consultations often over-run and this may have adverse effects for the GP. May need to agree to deal with some issues today, leaving others for later.

Patient issues

- Why does she want a referral? Have her previous consultations been unrewarding?
- What are her ideas, concerns and expectations? Does she think the rash is occupational? Is she hoping for compensation or to retire on medical grounds due to an occupational condition?
- Why did she go to the walk-in centre rather than the GP as a first step?
- Is she trying to play off the walk-in centre against the GP? Has she been refused a referral in the past?
- What would be the gain of a referral for her? Confirmation of allergy, allowing allergen avoidance?
- What are drawbacks of a referral? If the tests are negative how would she feel? What would she do?
- Are there any other problems in her life, eg marital difficulties or desperation to leave her job?

Doctor issues

- Acknowledge own feelings, eg irritation at demanding patients or walk-in centre which may prejudice approach to the patient.
- Conflict of interest between role as patient's advocate and gatekeeper for secondary care.
- Acknowledge own limitations in allergy and occupational medicine, and be prepared to refer if beyond these limitations.
- Any learning need?

Issues for society

- Walk-in centres: Do the public find second opinions independent of their GP helpful or confusing?
- Should nurses with computers be advising patients to ask for secondary care referrals? Do they just allow patients to manipulate the system, playing GPs off against the walk-in centre and vice versa?
- Is the benefits system a disincentive to work?

Management of the problem

- Acknowledge problem and review history.
- Definite pattern of allergy. What treatments have been tried? Is it purely occupational or does it occur at home? Can she take steps to avoid exposure at work?
- Examine patient. Is the rash typically allergic? Any evidence of other cause, eg SLE?
- Explain diagnosis in simple terms. Explain therapeutic options, eg start with non-sedating antihistamines, gloves, barrier or steroid creams. Offer trial of treatment for one month and refer if no better.
- Explain role of allergy testing, including chance of negative results. Acknowledge that proved allergy may suggest an occupational component, but explain implications, eg need to change jobs.
- Agree a mutually acceptable management plan, eg trial of non-sedating antihistamine for one month and refer if no better.
- Offer early consultation to review or reinforce information.
- Review call report from walk-in centre. Was the outcome as reported? Is there a problem with walk-in centre advice? Consider feedback, either positive or negative.
- Ideally recharge before next patient, eg with a cup of tea, if at all possible.
- If you feel the consultation has gone badly, discuss with partners or Balint group.

Answer 11

1   **With reference to recent literature, discuss the role of nurse practitioners in primary care.**

The NHS Plan described the intention to extend the role of nurses and to encourage all professionals to work together. Nurse practitioners have been seen as an ideal solution to manpower shortages in General Practice.

2   **Are nurse practitioners effective for chronic disease management?**

- A systematic review in 2002 in the *British Medical Journal*[1] suggests patients are more satisfied with care from a nurse practitioner than from a doctor, with no difference in health outcomes.
- Nurse practitioners provide longer consultations and carry out more investigations than doctors.
- Most recent research has related to patients requesting same day

appointments for minor illness, which is only a limited part of a doctor's role.

- Some of the trials are of questionable relevance to the NHS since qualifications and roles vary much throughout the world, as does the use of the term 'nurse practitioner'.
- An editorial in the *British Medical Journal* in 2000 [2] concluded that on average, nurses have longer consultations, arrange more investigations and follow-up, provide more information and give more satisfaction than GPs.
- Primary care nurses are not cheaper than GPs, but they are as safe in managing self-limiting illnesses.
- A trial [3] in the east end of London found that asthma specialist nurses running clinics and education medical staff reduced unscheduled care for asthma in a deprived multiethnic health district. However, not all ethnic groups benefited equally from specialist nurse intervention.
- A second trial [4] looking at education and facilitation by specialist nurses for primary care management of UTI in children improved the management of UTIs, was valued by doctors and parents, and may have prevented some renal scarring.
- Trials [5] looking at adding nurse practitioners to general practice teams and measuring workload in chronic disease areas, found that this did not reduce the workload of GPs, at least in the short term.
- This implies that nurse practitioners are used as supplements, rather than substitutes, for care given by GPs.

3   Are they useful for emergency appointments?

- When same day appointments were analysed [6] the clinical care and health service costs of nurse practitioners and GPs were similar. The authors concluded that if nurse practitioners were able to maintain the benefits while reducing their return consultation rate or shortening consultation times, they could be more cost-effective than GPs.

4   Are they useful for telephone triage?

- A trial [7] looking at workload over a 12-month period covering the introduction of nurse telephone triage found that this reduced the number of same-day appointments with GPs but resulted in busier routine surgeries, increased nursing time, and a small but significant increase in out-of-hours and A&E attendance.
- Lattimer [8] looked at nurse triage in out-of-hours care. Nurse telephone consultation halved the number of cases dealt with by GPs and was at least as safe as existing out-of-hours services. Nurse

telephone consultation replacing telephone advice given by a doctor led to reductions in both home visits and surgery attendances out of hours.

5   Are nurse minor illness clinics effective?

- In an RCT [9] in 73% of consultations no doctor input was needed. Again, patients were more satisfied with their consultations with nurses than their consultations with doctors.
- Clinical outcomes were similar among patients seen by nurses and those seen by doctors, and nurses took an average of eight minutes per patient compared with 10 minutes for GPs.

References

1   Systematic review of whether nurse practitioners working in primary care can provide equivalent care to doctors. *British Medical Journal* 2002; 324: 819–823

2   Nursing and the future of primary care [editorial]. *British Medical Journal* 2000; 320: 1020–1021

3   Specialist nurse intervention to reduce unscheduled asthma care in a deprived multiethnic area: the east London randomised controlled trial for high risk asthma (ELECTRA). *British Medical Journal* 2004; 328:144

4   A nurse led education and direct access service for the management of urinary tract infections in children: prospective controlled trial. *British Medical Journal* 2003; 327: 656

5   Impact of nurse practitioners on workload of general practitioners: randomised controlled trial. *British Medical Journal* 2004; 328: 927

6   Randomised controlled trial comparing cost effectiveness of general practitioners and nurse practitioners in primary care. *British Medical Journal* 2000; 320: 1048–1053

7   Nurse telephone triage for same day appointments in general practice: multiple interrupted time series trial of effect on workload and costs. *British Medical Journal* 2002; 325: 1214

8   Safety and effectiveness of nurse telephone consultation in out of hours primary care: randomised controlled trial. *British Medical Journal* 1998; 317: 1054–1059

9   Nurse management of patients with minor illnesses in general practice: multicentre, randomised controlled trial. *British Medical Journal* 2000; 320: 1038–1043

Answer 12

With reference to the literature discuss recent developments in the diagnosis and treatment of coughs and colds.

There are two aspects of management of respiratory tract infection in primary care: initial diagnosis and triage, and appropriate treatment and realistic prognosis.

- Evidence suggests GPs correctly predict the type of pathogen only 50% of the time [1] and often prescribe antibiotics knowing they will be ineffective [2].
- Attempts have been made to predict at initial presentation which patients are at risk of developing lower respiratory tract infection [3]. It was concluded that dry cough, diarrhoea, nausea, general impression of moderate or severe illness, temperature >38° C and chills were predictive of pneumonia. Purulent sputum, dyspnoea or auscultation findings were not found to be predictors of bacterial infection. CRP, with a high cut-off value of 20 mg/l, had a high predictive value for bacterial infection.
- Systematic reviews [4] and a prospective cohort study of 223 children with acute cough [5] have found a 10–12% complication rate which included persistent cough, but only three patients experienced serious complications.
- In other studies, 58% of patients still had cough at 10 days and 29% had not returned to their usual activities [6]. Giving a realistic prognosis at initial presentation may help to avoid re-consultation.
- Where the likely diagnosis is viral, strategies to avoid prescribing may include deferred scripts for antibiotics [7] or advice leaflets which reiterate the advice given, and give further advice on symptoms or signs of note.
- Studies of deferred scripts in upper respiratory tract infection suggest up to 55% of patients given a deferred script do not use it [2].
- Where pneumonia is possible, as suggested by the BTS recommendations with regard to community acquired pneumonia in adults [8] the following signs are important in triage of adults: confusion, tachypnoea (respiratory rate >30), and low blood pressure.
- It is also recommended that out-of-hours GP services should use a pulse oximeter for detecting hypoxia. These patients should be considered for hospital admission. The first line antibiotic of choice – if indicated – should be amoxicillin (or a macrolide if penicillin sensitive).
- For children, the BTS guidelines suggest age as a good predictor of organism: the under 5s usually viral, older children most commonly *Streptococcus pneumoniae*, followed by mycobacteria. Important

signs are tachypnoea with respiratory rate > 50, grunting and
dehydration.
- First line antibiotic – where indicated – is amoxicillin in under 5s
  but macrolides in over 5s due to prevalence of mycobacteria in this
  age group.

References

1 Aetiology of respiratory tract infections: clinical assessment versus
  serological tests. *British Journal of General Practice* 2001; 51:
  998–1000

2 A randomised controlled trial of delayed antibiotic prescribing as
  a strategy for managing uncomplicated respiratory tract infection
  in primary care. *British Journal of General Practice* 2001; 51:
  200–205

3 Contributions of symptoms, signs, erythrocyte sedimentation rate
  and C-reactive protein to a diagnosis of pneumonia in acute lower
  respiratory tract infection. *British Journal of General Practice*
  2003; 53: 358–364

4 The natural history of acute cough in children aged 0–4 years in
  primary care: systematic review. *British Journal of General
  Practice* 2002; 52: 401–409

5 Predicting complications from acute cough in pre-school children
  in primary care: prospective cohort study. *British Journal of
  General Practice* 2003; 54: 9–14

6 Symptoms, signs and prescribing for acute lower respiratory tract
  illness. *British Journal of General Practice* 2001; 51: 177–82

7 Delayed prescriptions in primary care. *British Journal of General
  Practice* 2003; 53: 836–837

8 BTS guidelines of community acquired pneumonia. *Thorax* 2001;
  56(suppl IV)

Paper 6

Answer 1

You see a 31-year-old man who has a purulent urethral discharge. Outline your management.

Consultation style

- Potentially awkward consultation. Aim to be open, honest and non-judgemental.
- Compliance and follow-up critical and depend on patient feeling understood and supported.
- Questions should be unambiguous and simple. Avoid assumptions about sexuality.
- Avoid own feelings and prejudices, eg about promiscuity affecting consultation.
- Offer GUM referral: benefits of greater confidentiality, rapid on-the-spot diagnosis and better able to perform contact tracing.

History

- Take a full sexual history, including previous history of infections.
- How was the infection acquired?
- Any associated symptoms, eg dysuria, conjunctivitis, joint pain?
- Any special risks, eg sex with a prostitute, or in sub-Saharan Africa?
- Is he at risk of HIV?
- Explore health belief model. Understanding of STDs, treatment and follow-up.

Examination

- Examine genitalia.
- Urethral swabs for *Chlamydia* and standard culture.
- Consider rectal and throat swabs if any history of anal or oral sex.
- Evidence of other STDs, eg inguinal lymph nodes (lymphogranuloma venereum), ulcers (syphilis or herpes)?
- General examination for signs of other disease, eg hepatitis, or lymphadenopathy if HIV is a possibility.

Contact tracing

- Emphasise need for open and honest discussion with sexual contacts.
- Need for screening and treatment of partner to prevent re-infection in patient, infection of others or untreated disease in contacts.

Treatment

- If compliance likely to be poor, consider stat doses, eg azithromycin.
- If gonorrhoea likely give ciprofloxacin. Co-infection with *Chlamydia* common so have a low threshold for treating after taking swabs.
- Advice on safe sex and give condoms if appropriate. Advice on risk of re-infection if partner not treated.

Summarise

- Explain likely diagnosis and implications.
- Offer opportunity to ask questions: How does he feel about diagnosis? Does he acknowledge the diagnosis? Any preconceptions, eg I cannot get gonorrhoea because I have only had sex once in the last year. Only homosexuals get AIDS, etc.[Q24]
- Explain treatment and procedure for results of swabs sent.
- Arrange follow-up for results, and to discuss further tests, eg HIV, hepatitis.
- Offer written information about the issues covered and give information about GUM clinic.

Practice issues

- Check confidentiality policy regarding sensitive results, eg not to be given over phone, etc.
- Need for more health information regarding STDs, eg posters in waiting room?
- Is there a learning need for the GP/nurses, eg current guidelines for treatment?
- Is there a problem with access to GUM services? Consider raising with the PCT.
- Acknowledge own feelings after consultation, perhaps have a cup of tea before the next patient.

Answer 2

You are telephoned by the daughter of Mr Smith, an 81-year-old widower who lives alone. She lives in Canada and visits infrequently. She says that he is unsafe living alone and wants you to put him into a home. What issues does this raise?

This potentially difficult problem requires a sensitive, cautious approach, acknowledging the feelings and wishes of all involved.

Issues relating to the consultation

- Difficulties of telephone consultations, with lack of visual cues and pressures of cost of overseas calls.
- Be aware that the daughter lives in a country with a different healthcare system, where services and attitudes to autonomy may be different. This may require patient explanation; you should not assume that the daughter understands the system in the UK.

Issues relating to the daughter

- You risk breaching Mr Smith's confidentiality in discussions with the daughter. Even though she may be next of kin he still has the right to confidentiality. Explain that you can record her concerns and act on them but are unable to give medical details without consent.
- Ideas, concerns and expectations: What are her concerns? Any new symptoms that you were unaware of, eg falls? Is she aware of risky behaviour, eg heavy drinking? Have neighbours expressed concerns to her? What does she expect?
- Why has she telephoned now? Does she feel guilty because she is not caring for him?
- Any other motive for wanting him to go to a home, eg the sale of his property?
- Does she have enduring power of attorney over his affairs? If so, she may be able to make decisions for him.

Issues relating to Mr Smith

- Autonomy: Is he mentally competent? If so, he has the right to self-determination and removing him from his house would be an infringement of his human rights.
- Risk: Is he at risk, eg of falling, drinking too much? Is he able to look after himself?
- Is he depressed or lonely? Has his daughter picked this up, triggering her call?

- Has there been a change in his medical condition, eg heart failure that has rendered him bed-bound?
- Is he getting any help at home from family locally or social services?

Issues for the GP

- Acknowledge the daughter's concerns. It is easy to become irritated with absent relatives who make apparently unreasonable demands.
- Be prepared to reassess Mr Smith's medical, psychological and social situation, and act accordingly.
- Review record keeping, eg regarding next of kin, power of attorney, at-risk register for elderly.

Implications for the PHCT

- If Mr Smith is genuinely at risk, why has this not been picked up before?
- Does the practice need to be pro-active in care of elderly people, eg health visitor to carry out over-75 checks?
- Is there a problem with social services resources in the area?
- Any learning needs regarding rights of patients and relatives in this situation?

Answer 3

A 14-year-old boy comes to see you with his parents. He has just been discharged from hospital after having an epileptic seizure. What issues would you aim to cover and what would be your management aims?

This situation raises a number of issues both for the patient and his family, and for the practice. The aims of management are to minimise seizures and achieve a normal quality of life.

Consultation issues

- Do not hurry. Encourage everyone to contribute. Solicit his views particularly, without talking over him.
- Encourage them to take notes if they wish.
- Explore their beliefs about epilepsy and accommodate these.
- Bear in mind they may be going through a form of bereavement.
- Investigate their ideas, concerns and expectations? Do they blame themselves, eg for dropping him as a baby? Are they terrified it is genetic and thus want to avoid future pregnancies? Do they fear he will be mentally handicapped?

- What are his ideas, concerns and expectations? Driving, choice of career?

Medical issues

- Review history, including current working diagnosis. What have they been told?
- What future investigations and follow-up are planned?
- Review treatment: Is he being treated at present?
- Are they aware of side-effects of treatment, eg need to check blood levels? Drug interactions?
- Do they know what to do in event of another seizure?
- Agree treatment goals: Aim for minimal seizures, normal quality of life.
- Explain that if seizure-free on medication he may be able to stop his drugs and drive later.

Health and safety issues

- Explain need to avoid potentially dangerous sports, eg swimming alone.
- Advise the family about provoking factors and avoidance.
- Is there a need to educate school, eg what he can and cannot do?

Social issues

- Encourage him to be open with friends and family about his problem. Surveys suggest > 50% do not even tell their fiancées.
- Explain need to comply with medication and anticipate problems, eg with drinking, dancing, etc.
- Give written advice about support groups, eg British Epilepsy Association.

Practice issues

- Does the practice need to audit its care of people with epilepsy? Surveys suggest GP care is often substandard.
- Is there a need for a register, with appropriate follow-up and drug monitoring, ensuring compliance and identification of side-effects?
- Any learning needs?

Answer 4

> You practise in a busy urban practice with high deprivation scores. One of your partners announces at the practice meeting that he wants to become a trainer. What are the implications of his request?

This situation may arise for a number of reasons and affects the practice at many levels.

Implications for the partner who wishes to become a trainer

- Why does he want to be a trainer? Does he no longer find work fulfilling? Is this escapism?
- May enhance clinical skills and knowledge through teaching.
- Will need to go on trainers' course, resulting in time away from surgery and will lose one to two sessions a week through tutorials and joint surgeries when training.
- May find interruptions to surgery to help trainee disruptive and stressful.
- Will have burden of supervision and paperwork in addition to normal workload.
- Must be prepared to be challenged by trainee.

Implications for the practice

- Need to provide a room and secretarial time for trainee.
- Need to be aware of trainee's requirements (eg video consent forms), and be able to advise patients about the trainee and what they do.
- Practice facilities may need upgrading, eg installation of video camera.
- Staff need to know limitations of trainee, not to consider them as another partner.
- Need to ensure protected time for trainee, may need assistance with audit, etc.
- Will need adequate notices to inform patients, including practice leaflet.

Implications for partners

- Individual workload may be higher at first, due to loss of trainer's sessions and slow pace of a new trainee, but lower later.
- Trainee may need supervision when trainer is away.

- There may be concern about trainees being present at practice meetings.
- Need to clarify situation regarding out-of-hours care, to avoid resentment over whom the trainee does sessions for.
- Some financial benefit as trainee's salary paid by health authority and training grant payable to practice.
- Trainee more likely to make mistakes; partners need to be aware of this and compensate accordingly.
- Need ground rules regarding trainee, eg working unsupervised, particularly early on.

Implications for patients

- May lack confidence in trainee's skills/advice or relish the opportunity for fresh opinion.
- May be popular with certain patients, eg young women if the trainee is a woman.
- May be asked to participate in video surgeries. May not feel able to say no.
- May be concerned about confidentiality, particularly in video surgeries.
- May find joint surgeries awkward.
- May not understand difference between a medical student and a trainee. May abuse the trainee, eg for drug seeking or sick certification.
- Trainees often run behind, causing agitation for patients.

Answer 5

Reducing suicide is a national priority. Discuss the available evidence relating to primary care in this area.

This topic was covered in the April 2004 issue of the *British Journal of General Practice* (editorial and papers). Goldberg and Huxley[1] described three filters in care:

- the decision to consult and attend at primary care setting
- the recognition of a mental health problem and appropriate management
- onward referral from primary care.

Primary care is involved in the first and second filters. People at risk presenting to primary care depends on whether they can acknowledge that a problem exists and whether they are able to express this to a primary care professional.

- A retrospective survey of suicides[2] demonstrated 68% had clear evidence of mental illness in the month before death, suggesting that recognising and dealing appropriately with this may reduce the frequency of suicide.

- Other studies have shown that over 60% men with severe depression had not seen their GP in the last year [3], and studies of suicides among young men [4] show that relatively few had seen their GP in the three months before death.

- A study of health-seeking behaviour in young men when mentally disturbed [5] found that they were particularly unlikely to seek help unless they were severely distressed. They did not seek lay support. This gender-specific pattern may explain why men are more likely to commit suicide whereas women are more likely to self-harm.

- To improve care at filter one, we need to improve presentation of mentally distressed patients to primary care. The increase in options available to people with advent of NHS Direct and walk-in centres will help. It offers potential 24-hour access in an anonymous setting, however, long queues at walk-in centres and waiting for callbacks may be a disincentive.

- Young men do not present frequently to primary care, due to inconvenient access for patients who work, and when depressed this group of men typically cope through exercise, alcohol or drugs rather than seeking help. Women tend to confide in friends and family [6].

- It may help to publicise the range of choices for access, encouraging people with physical and mental health issues to attend, eg through posters or practice leaflets, convenient surgery times and opportunistic advice, eg when patients attend for travel vaccination.

- Once patients have attended, one needs to recognise and act on the problems. Historically, studies have shown that GPs do not recognise depression very well. However, a study of 100 suicides in Devon [2] found that recognition of mental health problems was much better than previously reported, but that suicide risk assessments were only recorded in 15% of cases.

- We need to look for warning signs, such as gender, age and substance abuse. Angst [6] found that symptoms may differ between the sexes, with men having fewer classic symptoms.

- We need a lower threshold of diagnosis in these groups. Suicides are relatively rare in general practice, with the average GP seeing one every four to seven years. Any suicides or attempted suicides should be treated as significant events (they are as part of the nGMS contract) and lessons looked for.

- The second and third filters depend on local resources. Where there is a long wait for traditional secondary care services should the

practice or PCT look at local initiatives, eg on-call CPN service, crisis resolution team that will make telephone contact and give support?
- You may need to educate staff and health workers about mental health and avoiding unhelpful stereotypes and stigmas. Consider away-day training to improve detection and treatment.

References

1 Goldberg D, Huxley P. *Common Mental Disorders. A biosocial model*. London: Tavistock/Routledge, 1992
2 Owens C, Lloyd KR, Campbell J. Access to health care prior to suicide: findings from a psychological autopsy study. *British Journal of General Practice* 2004; 54: 279–281
3 Bebbington PE, Meltzer H, Brugha TS et al. Unequal access and unmet need: neurotic disorders and the use of primary care services. *Psychological Medicine* 2000; 30: 1359–1367
4 Stanistreet D, Gabbay MB, Jeffrey V, Taylor S. Missed opportunities? Preventing violent deaths in young men, an epidemiological study. *British Journal of General Practice* 2004; 54: 254–258
5 Biddle L, Gunnell D, Sharp D, Donovan JL. Factors influencing health seeking in mentally distressed young adults: a cross sectional survey. *British Journal of General Practice* 2004; 54: 248–253
6 Angst J, Gamma A, Gastpar M, Lepine J-P, Mendlewicz J, Tylee A. Gender differences in depression. Epidemiological findings from the European DEPRES I and II studies. *European Archives of Psychiatry and Clinical Neuroscience* 2002; 252: 201–209

Answer 6

What are the difficulties when dealing with patients who abuse opiate drugs?

The DOH sees primary care as the ideal setting for treatment of drug abuse. There are a number of potential problems in caring for these patients.

Problems for the patient

- Does the patient know how to contact the doctor and use the appointment system?
- Chaotic lifestyle may cause difficulties attending for appointments.
- Prejudice: attitudes of previous doctors and reception staff (eg

removal from list) may alienate or impede rapport.
- Social circumstances: lack of support or family guidance can hinder healthcare. Drugs users are more likely to be unemployed, have a history of crime and live in poor housing. May be malnourished.
- Drug users are less likely to be offered preventive healthcare by the practice, and they are less likely to take it up.

Problems during the consultation

- Rapport: engage the patient and allow respect for autonomy. Avoid adopting a parental role. Involve the patient in decisions.
- You may be biased by past experiences with drug abusers or perceive pressure to prescribe. Address problems at face value. Addicts often present in a crisis or with complex or difficult requests.
- Safety: consider a position near the door if there is a risk of violence. Is there a panic alarm?
- Consider a treatment plan or contract with the patient. This needs to be explicit and agreed early, eg not attending when drunk/under influence of drugs, always to see same doctor.
- Make explicit rules if you agree to prescribe drugs, eg no lost scripts/early scripts.
- Social issues: are there 'at-risk' children or partner. Are there any court cases pending?
- Seek mental health or other medical problems, eg sepsis, heart murmurs.
- Consider contacting previous doctor/drugs services for previous history. Shared care, eg with drugs services, can lead to the problems of manipulation or repetition.
- Is there a need for urinary screening for drugs?

Problems for the practice

- Practice policy: practices sometimes refuse all intravenous drug abusers as regular patients, in which case they need to be directed to an appropriate source of medical care.
- Consider a named doctor always to see patient for continuity of care and to avoid manipulation. May need to ensure patients see a partner rather than a registrar or locum.
- Prescribing policy: do the doctors prescribe methadone? If so, is this under the support or guidance of the local specialist drug team? Risks of prescribing in patients who still inject.
- Contracts: the receptionists need to know which patients are being seen under 'contract' and what the contract entails, eg only to see a particular doctor.

- Staff safety: all staff need to know about violent patients. Mark notes as high risk, or put alert message on the computer.
- Staff concerns and prejudice: allow staff to express concerns at meetings and formulate solutions.
- HIV/hepatitis risk: consider marking notes as high risk. Ideally the patient should be informed.
- Notification of addicts is encouraged by the DOH.
- Workload implications: may attract other drug abusers. The average addict undergoing treatment has been shown to consult up to 32 times per year.
- Funding: if large numbers of addicts, approach PCT for funding. Possible PMS contract.
- Security: consider risks of prescription fraud, etc.

Ethical considerations

- Justice: All patients should be treated fairly with respect to medical care.
- Autonomy: Patient's right to choose lifestyle. GP's right to autonomy on prescribing decisions.
- Beneficence: Avoid inflicting harm or failing to prevent harm, eg not providing necessary care.
- Non-maleficence: Offer choices in their care and to minimise risk of harm, eg prescribing methadone inappropriately.

Answer 7

Outline ways in which practices can improve access for disabled patients.

We have a moral and legal duty to ensure practices provide adequate access for disabled patients, and this may take several forms.

Assess current situation

- Consider the skills base within the practice staff, eg lip reading.
- Consider the range of disabilities likely to be encountered now and in the future, eg physical, intellectual, impaired hearing, vision or speech?
- What facilities already exist?
- Involve all the staff for a broad perspective on problems and possible improvements.
- Does the practice leaflet include access for disabled people? Is it clear and suitable, eg Braille?

- Audit access: Disabled parking? Wide doorways and disabled toilets? Wheelchair ramps or lifts if consulting upstairs?

Premises improvements

- Consider outreach clinics, eg local schools for disabled people, with doctor seeing patients in familiar surroundings or scheduled visits to local nursing homes.
- Clearly visible signs, eg large font.
- Consider Braille on important signs and notices within the surgery.
- If there is a call system, can patients hear or see it? Consider an induction loop for hearing aids.
- Privacy for hard of hearing: Is there a soundproofed area for giving results or talking to receptionist?

Improving staff skills

- Staff training should include appreciation of problems experienced by disabled patients.
- Respect for autonomy, patience and sensitivity are essential when dealing with patients.
- Doctor–patient relationship enhanced if patients feel their problems are being understood.
- Consider the patient's mental capacity. Can they understand appointment times?

Other issues

- Clarify the carer's position and role – mental advocate or assistant with mobility? Carers' register should be established. What are their needs?
- Patient's autonomy should be respected and the patient involved in decisions where possible.
- Consider patient's confidentiality, establish whether they wish the carer to be present and what information may be shared with them.
- Patients group should have disabled representatives.
- Any useful ideas from other practices?
- Look at links and involvement of social services, financially and for practical support.
- Is there any funding available from the local primary care organisation?

Answer 8

What do current guidelines suggest regarding the following areas of management of hypertension:

1 Initial assessment

- British Hypertension Society guidelines[1] suggest initial assessment to confirm diagnosis, exclude secondary hypertension and evaluate end-organ damage.
- Diagnosis should not be based on one reading.
- Investigations should include urine strip test for protein and blood, serum creatinine and electrolytes, glucose, fasting lipids and ECG. These data can then be used to calculate the 10-year cardiac risk.
- Ambulatory BP recording is useful in evaluating unusual variability of blood pressure, white-coat hypertension, nocturnal hypertension (which may be associated with early diabetes), drug-resistant hypertension, diagnosis and treatment of hypertension in pregnancy and evaluation of symptomatic hypotension. The NICE guidelines[2] do not recommend routine use of ambulatory blood pressure monitoring.

2 Treatment

- BHF guidelines suggest all patients should be given lifestyle advice, eg moderate intake of alcohol, smoking, salt intake, exercise and weight loss[3].
- Patients with grade I hypertension (BP 140–159/90–99 mmHg) should be considered for treatment if they have other risk factors, eg diabetes or end-organ damage. If they do not, a trial of six months lifestyle treatment should be undertaken.
- Patients with grade II hypertension (BP >160/100 mmHg) should be started on treatment according to the AB/CD rule (see Figure overleaf). NICE guidelines suggest a different approach, starting with a low-dose thiazide, then adding a β-blocker or an ACE-inhibitor if the patient is at risk of diabetes. Calcium channel blockers are considered third-line drugs.
- The NICE guidelines suggest that patients over the age of 80 years should be treated in the same way as those under 80 years. Once daily drugs should be used where possible.

3 Statins/aspirin

- Ten-year risk should be calculated for all patients. Where this is > 20% the Heart Protection[4] and ASCOT[5] studies suggest statins

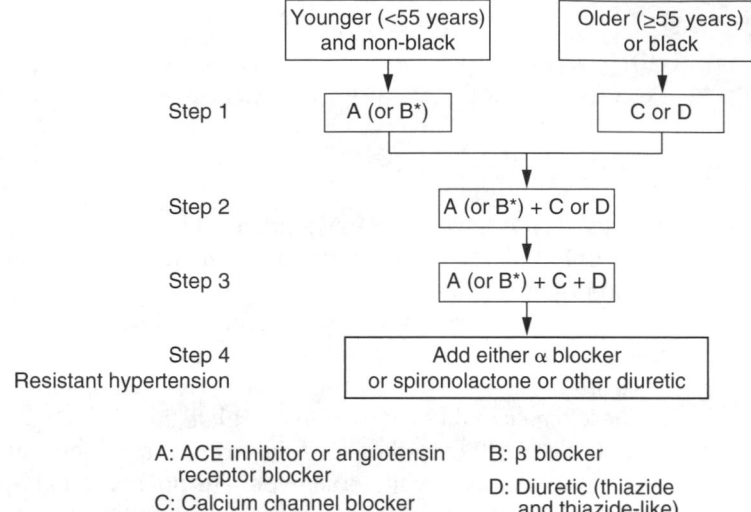

A: ACE inhibitor or angiotensin receptor blocker

B: β blocker

C: Calcium channel blocker

D: Diuretic (thiazide and thiazide-like)

and aspirin are of benefit, respectively.
* New ideal targets are: Lower total cholesterol by 25% or LDL cholesterol by 30% or reach < 4.0 mmol/L or < 2.0 mmol/L, respectively, whichever is greater.
* The NICE guidelines also suggest a cut-off of 20% cardiovascular risk for statin/aspirin use.

References

1   British Hypertension Society guidelines for hypertension management 2004 (BHS-IV): summary. *British Medical Journal* 2004; 328: 634–640

2   Hypertension. Management of hypertension in adults in primary care. NICE CG18, August 2004

3   DASH – Sodium Collaborative Research Group. Effects on blood pressure of reduced dietary sodium and the dietary approaches to stop hypertension (DASH) diet. *New England Journal of Medicine* 2001; 344: 3–10

4   MRC/BHF heart protection study of cholesterol lowering with simvastatin in 20 536 high-risk individuals: a randomised placebo-controlled trial. *The Lancet* 2002; 360: 7–22

5   Prevention of coronary and stroke events with atorvastatin in hypertensive patients who have average or lower-than average cholesterol concentrations, in the Anglo Scandinavian Cardiac Outcomes Trial-Lipid Lowering Arm (ASCOT-LLA): A multicentre randomised controlled trial. *The Lancet* 2003; 361: 1149–1158

Answer 9

> Mr Jones, who has complained of impotence since being treated for a heart attack, asks for a prescription for sildenafil (Viagra), which you have not previously prescribed. You agree to look into it and come across an article entitled 'Systematic review of randomised controlled trials of sildenafil (Viagra) in the treatment of male erectile dysfunction' (reprinted with permission by *British Journal of General Practice* 2001; 51: 1004 – 1012; reference material 6.1a).

1   Comment on the selection process used

- The researchers sought to identify all published and unpublished randomised controlled trials. The electronic and hand searches were thorough, together with further searches of references in the identified papers. This should identify all relevant published trials.
- The description is not specific as to how unpublished trials were sought. It may be that Pfizer has omitted to provide unpublished trials showing lack of effect, ie inclusion bias towards trials showing effect.
- Assessment of quality was undertaken by two independent researchers. This should help to minimise inclusion bias.

2   Comment on the trials identified (see Table 1 in reference material 6.1b)

- The search identified 20 trials with 4000 participants, including a broad range of aetiologies such as spinal cord damage, diabetes and idiopathic erectile dysfunction. This large number, together with the long follow-up of six months, should give an adequate sample population.
- Exclusion criteria were broad with a lot of exclusions which may limit the generalisability of the study to a general practice population.
- Data on withdrawals was not reported, which is unfortunate since the side-effect profile is clinically relevant, but the analysis was done on an intention-to-treat basis.

3   Comment on the endpoints used

The endpoints were clinically relevant, and used a standardised system. Secondary endpoints were also included for some studies, such as quality-of-life questionnaires and partner questionnaires, which gives an indication of overall acceptability.

4   Comment on the results in Figure 1 in reference material 6.1c and their applicability to Mr Jones

- These studies all show a statistically significant effect of sildenafil in the Global Efficacy question 'Did treatment improve your erections?' The confidence intervals for individual studies are all in the positive zone favouring treatment, and the Forest plot shows that the combined results give a risk difference of 0.537 with narrow confidence intervals of 0.484-0.589. This suggests an NNT of 2.
- Mr Jones has IHD and thus would have been excluded from these studies. For this reason it is not possible to extrapolate these data regarding safety or efficacy to him.

Answer 10

With reference to the literature, discuss the evidence for and against the following areas of prostate cancer management:

1   Diagnosis

- PSA testing can detect early disease, but many of these will not cause problems if untreated [1].
- Sensitivity and specificity low: Using a cut-off of 4 ng/ml 13% of cases will be missed but go on to develop cancer in the next four years [2]. A study of biopsies in symptomatic men showed cancer in 11% of men with PSA < 4ng/ml [3].
- Digital rectal examination has similar problems of sensitivity and specificity [4], so most people advocate a combination of DRE and PSA testing, with positives being referred for biopsy.

2   Treatment

Main dilemma is whether to watch and wait or treat actively.

Conservative treatment

Watchful waiting

- No initial treatment, 6–12 monthly evaluation for symptoms of metastasis.
- Palliative hormonal therapy given to patients with significant symptoms. NICE [4] recommends for older patients with co-morbidity and well-differentiated cancer (more likely to die with than from their cancer).
- Studies [5] estimate a man aged 70–74 years in this group would

have a 7% chance of dying within 15 years from his cancer but a 73% chance of dying from other causes in this time.

Active surveillance

- Three monthly clinical review and PSA/DRE. If PSA rises repeatedly offered radical treatment while disease still potentially curable.

Active treatment

- Radical prostatectomy: May reduce risk of metastatic disease and death by 50% [6]. 60% patients are impotent and up to 33% incontinent.
- External beam radiotherapy: For patients with PSA < 10 and Gleason score < 6, 5-year survival of 85% [1]. 50% patients are impotent, 12% have radiation proctitis and 7% incontinent with standard external beam radiotherapy, less so with conformal radiotherapy (matching irradiated volume to tumour volume) [7].
- Brachytherapy: Radioactive pellets implanted under ultrasound guidance, achieves therapeutic dosage of radiotherapy locally with minimal damage to other pelvic organs. Cannot be used if previous TURP. Minimal long-term outcome data. Side-effects include increased frequency, retention and nocturia, however, after three months incidence of these side-effects is 1 – 2% [8]. Impotence affects 40%.

Hormone therapy

- Effective for advanced forms of cancer, or in combination for early disease.
- Bicalutamide causes increased mortality so Committee on Safety of Medicines recommend not to use.
- Side-effects include hot flushes, impotence, weight gain, gynaecomastia, osteoporosis.

Combination therapy

- There are no long-term outcome data on prostatectomy plus radiotherapy, prostatectomy plus hormone treatment, brachytherapy plus external beam radiotherapy or hormone treatment and radiotherapy.

References

1 Management of localised prostate cancer. *Drug Therapy Bulletin* 2004; 42: 81 – 84

2 Test sensitivity of prostate specific antigen in the Finnish randomised prostate cancer screening trial. *International Journal of Cancer* 2004; 111: 940–943

3 Measurement of prostate specific antigen in serum as a screening test for prostate cancer. *New England Journal of Medicine* 1991:324;1156–61

4 National Institute of Clinical Excellence. Guidance on Cancer Services. Improving outcomes in urological cancers. www.nice.org.uk

5 Competing risk analysis of men aged 55 to 74 years at diagnosis managed conservatively for clinically localised prostate cancer. *Journal of the American Medical Association* 1998; 280: 975–980

6 A randomised controlled trial comparing radical prostatectomy with watchful waiting in early waiting in early prostate cancer. *New England Journal of Medicine* 2002; 347: 781–9

7 Comparison of radiation side effects of conformal and conventional radiotherapy in prostate cancer: a randomised trial. *The Lancet* 1999; 353: 267–272

8 Quality of life following treatment for early prostate cancer: does low dose rate (LDR) brachytherapy offer a better outcome? A review. *European Urology* 2004; 45: 134–141

Answer 11

Your practice is looking at designing a protocol for the management of blood pressure in the nurse-led diabetic clinic. You wish the process to be evidence-based. See reference material 4.2a, an extract from the paper 'Tight blood pressure control and risk of macrovascular and microvascular complications in type 2 diabetes: UK PDS 38' (with copyright permission from *British Medical Journal* 1998; 317: 703–713).

1 **Comment on the strengths and weaknesses of the methodology**

- The study had a focused research question: to determine whether tight control reduced complications.
- The population were recruited from general practice but managed in hospital outpatients, which may reduce generalisability to primary care.
- The inclusion criteria included fasting plasma glucose > 6 mmol/l on two consecutive mornings. This is lower than the WHO diagnostic criteria and may have resulted in misdiagnosis of normal patients or those with impaired glucose tolerance rather than type 2 diabetes.
- Patients who could not take β blockers (ie could not safely be

randomised), or those who had a requirement for strict blood
pressure control were excluded. These are reasonable exclusion
criteria since it would be unethical to randomise patients to less
strict control that might harm them.
- Randomisation produced baseline characteristics that were
  essentially similar in every respect except for visual acuity, which
  was significantly worse in the less tight treatment group. The ethnic
  mix was the same, which is important as different ethnic groups
  respond differently to certain drugs.
- The treatment protocol used a target BP of 200/105 mmHg but this
  was reduced half way through the trial. This may bias the results in
  favour of tight control, since damage may have been done in terms
  of complications before the change to lower limits.

2   Comment on the results shown in Figure 4 (reference material
    6.2b)

- There is a statistically significant reduction in any diabetes-related
  endpoint, deaths related to diabetes, microvascular complications
  and stroke, all with p values < 0.05.
- The confidence intervals are wide, however, and approach the line
  of no effect.
- The absolute risk reductions are 16% for all endpoints, 6% for
  deaths related to diabetes, 7% for microvascular disease and 5% for
  stroke.
- This represents NNT of 6, 16, 16 and 20 to prevent each of these
  endpoints.

3   Comment on the overall validity of the results

- Studies of ACE inhibitors have shown that these have a beneficial
  effect on vasculature independent of their antihypertensive
  properties. The system of allocating patients to either tight control
  with ACE inhibitors or loose control without, may mean that it is not
  the tight blood pressure control but the ACE inhibitor that is
  responsible.
- Comparing tight control with any drug combination to loose control
  with any drug combination would have answered this question.
- In particular, the finding that stroke is less common in the tight
  control group may be due to this effect, since the HOPE study has
  shown that stroke is reduced in patients on ramipril despite a mean
  blood pressure reduction of only 3/2 mmHg.
- The endpoints for retinal photocoagulation are potentially
  subjective and this combined with the difference in visual acuities
  between the two groups may have introduced bias.

- The baseline characteristics in terms of treatment of diabetes are given at randomisation, but not at the end of the trial. Patients within the tight control group could have had different treatments for diabetes, eg higher use of insulin, which may have been confounding.

4   Comment on the generalisability of the results to general practice

- The patients were not all diabetic by conventional WHO criteria, since the cut-off used was fasting plasma glucose of 6 mmol/l, so the results may not be applicable to care of all diabetics.
- Patients were followed-up in the hospital outpatient setting which may bring better blood pressure control than general practice-based treatment. Similarly, there may be an exaggerated 'white-coat' hypertension response at hospital compared with general practice, giving even tighter control as a result.

Answer 12

Your practice is attempting to shorten access times to comply with government targets. One of the areas you decide to concentrate on is frequent attenders. See reference material 6.3a, an extract from 'Psychosocial, lifestyle, and health status variables in predicting high attendance among adults' (with copyright permission from *British Journal of General Practice* 2001; 51: 987-994).

1   Comment on the strengths and weaknesses of the methodology

Strengths

- Clear aims, study design appropriate in attempting to answer the question.
- Study carried out in metropolitan UK, covering all practices within a 30-mile radius of the administrative centre. This makes it less prone to inclusion bias.
- The postal questionnaire method gives a good cross-sectional coverage, but relies on good records from GPs of up-to-date addresses.
- The questionnaire used validated indices to get objective assessments of various factors, allowing comparison between different groups.
- The sample size was calculated before the study, and the number of participants exceeded the calculation, which should give the study

sufficient power.
- The statistical analysis was specified in the paper and is a validated method.
- Respondents were compared with national statistics to test whether they are representative of the country as a whole.
- The questionnaire responses were validated by comparing self-reported attendance with medical records for a sample of patients.

Weaknesses

- The administrative centre is not specified; it may be in the area of Southampton around the university with socio-demographic characteristics not typical of the city as a whole. Within that area there were only six general practices. This suggests either low population density or large multi-doctor practices. These may not be representative of inner city or rural practices.
- Written questionnaires are less likely to be filled out by those whose first language is not English, who are illiterate or who have visual problems. All of these are potentially high users of services.
- Using a postal questionnaire together with information leaflets for another study may lead participants to feel they are being criticised about their attendance, and those with high attendances may not respond. It might have been better to use the questionnaire on all patients attending surgery.
- Not including those over 80 years or in nursing homes, and children, removes a large percentage of frequent attenders. Information on these patients is important in analysing workload.

2   Comment on the results given in Tables 2 and 4 of reference material 6.3b

- These show statistically significant associations with female sex and no academic qualifications (p values 0.006 and < 0.001, respectively).
- None of the other associations in Table 2 is statistically significant.
- In Table 4 there are statistically significant associations with medically unexplained symptoms (p = 0.006), health anxiety (p = 0.001), perceived health (p < 0.001), lack of negative attitudes to doctors (p < 0.001) and not trying the pharmacist first (p < 0.001). Low alcohol use is associated with attendance (p = 0.002).

3   Suggest possible interventions based on these results

- Measures to try to combat health anxiety and perceived health, eg

CBT, may be appropriate in reducing attendance.

- Tackling medically unexplained symptoms is difficult and therapies such as CBT may be more expensive in terms of resources and time than the savings to be made in reduced attendance.
- Encouraging more use of the pharmacist may not be effective if the people who attend the doctor first have psychological or complex needs that cannot be addressed by a consultation with a pharmacist. Transferring large quantities of work to pharmacists may result in them charging for this service, negating any savings made.

Paper 7

Answer 1

A local headmaster with type 2 diabetes refuses to take medication, preferring homoeopathic treatment. He refuses to attend the diabetic clinic. Bloods show a fasting blood sugar of 12, HbA1c 9.6, BP 184/102, BMI 36. How would you manage his care?

This situation requires tact and patience to ensure a mutually acceptable outcome. The GP should aim to have an open consulting style that actively solicits and acknowledges the patient's thoughts and feelings. He is a professional man and will expect to be treated accordingly.

Review history

- Explain diagnosis, relate to any symptoms he may have.
- Explore health beliefs: knowledge of diabetes, treatment and complications.
- Worried that he will have to give up driving if he admits he is diabetic?
- Worried that he may lose his job and income? Terrified of injections?
- Explore feelings about diagnosis. Does he believe he has diabetes? Try to answer his questions. Does he fear stigma of chronic disease?
- Any family history of note, eg ischaemic heart disease?
- Any confounding factors, eg steroids giving false positive results?
- Discuss events since diagnosis. Did he refuse to attend the nurse-led clinic because of denial, inconvenient timing or because he did not want to be seen by a nurse? Genuine belief in alternative medicine or denial?
- Does he accept the diagnosis? Did he experience unacceptable drug side-effects eg diarrhoea from metformin, that led him to homoeopathy?

Examination and investigations

- Examine for complications and co-morbidity. Test urine for protein and blood pressure (nephropathy), visual acuity, BMI, evidence of

neuropathy.
• Arrange ECG. Check fasting lipids.

Explain the findings

• Explain diagnosis and presence and relevance of any complications. Give realistic prognosis. Aim of treatment is normal quality of life and a normal life expectancy (St Vincent Declaration).
• Explain planned treatment and importance of lifestyle (healthy diet, exercise, smoking and ideal weight).
• Explain how the practice manages diabetes. Offer choice of nurse-led clinic or GP. Importance of retinal screening.
• Explain the implications of diagnosis. He must inform the DVLA and car insurers. Eligible for free prescriptions, if on drug therapy.
• Give written information, including the British Diabetic Association.

Agree treatment goals and plan treatment

• Realistic goals. Start with lifestyle, ie diet, exercise. Consider dietician referral.
• Aim for monthly reviews at convenient time if possible. Offer early review or telephone advice.
• Promote nurse-led clinic. Evidence suggests better routine care.
• If he fails to respond, he will need drug treatment, ideally with metformin initially, together with control of his blood pressure (UKPDS).
• If there are complications, consider referral to an endocrinologist.
• Consider writing to homoeopath to ensure care is complementary rather than antagonistic.
• Ensure the patient is on the diabetes register.
• Consider initial hospital referral for advice/reinforcement of message.

Review case at next PHCT meeting

• Do patients have a problem attending diabetic clinics?
• Is everyone consistent in their diagnosis of diabetes? Does everyone know the latest diagnostic criteria?
• Any learning needs, eg when to use insulin?
• Are many patients turning to complementary medicine? If so, does this reflect a problem with the service patients are getting?

Answer 2

> Following an audit by the GP registrar it has been brought to
> your attention as trainer that one of the senior partners has
> been prescribing excessive amounts of benzodiazepines. What
> issues does this raise?

Frequent prescribing of benzodiazepines is discouraged because of
problems of addiction, tolerance, withdrawal and risk of falls in the
elderly.

Issues relating to the audit

- Why was it done? After a significant event?
- Was this issue already known to be a problem within the practice,
  and an audit performed by a temporary member of staff such as the
  GP registrar seen as a good way of bringing it into the open?
- Who initiated the audit – the registrar? Or a partner/trainer?
- Danger of audit being seen as an underhand way of investigating
  one person's practice.
- Was everyone in the practice aware that an audit was taking place?
- How was the audit conducted – across the practice or only
  involving certain partners? Was the methodology used accurate and
  the conclusions drawn appropriate?

Issues for the registrar

- The topic of the audit and the results obtained could cause
  difficulties for the partner identified. They could feel like a
  scapegoat.
- Are they uncomfortable about bringing such information into the
  open?
- How does it affect their relationship with the partner concerned?
  May result in interpersonal difficulties or avoidance.
- May affect interactions with other practice staff, eg may not trust the
  registrar.
- May worry about future job prospects if widely known to be a
  'trouble maker'.

Issues for the trainer

- Responsible not only for the practice patients and staff but also for
  the wellbeing and support of registrar.
- The situation may represent a conflict of interest.
- Not only need to deal appropriately with the information, putting
  the safety of patients first (following GMC guidelines), but also need

to deal sensitively with the partner concerned.
- Consider involving practice manager, possible meeting in private with partner concerned to discuss audit and look for causes.
- Should the results of the audit be presented anonymously or be completely open? Who should attend? Partners and practice manager or other staff?
- Agree rules, eg significant event-type session without blame.
- Consider seeking advice from LMC/protection societies.

Issues for the senior partner

- Why are they prescribing so much? May be legitimate, eg many psychiatric patients, drug users or patients withdrawing from alcohol.
- Prescriptions could have been initiated by specialists or by a previous doctor, ie patients on this medication for many years and unable or not prepared to stop.
- Does this identify a need for education? Eg of risks of benzodiazepines and alternatives available, or methods of treating addiction and services available to help.
- Other areas of their practice might also be dangerous. Do they need a full review of practice/re-education?
- Could this be prescription fraud with illegal selling of benzodiazepines?
- Could they have medical problems, eg alcohol/drug misuse, and be self-medicating? This audit may be the catalyst needed for him to admit the problem and seek help.
- Is this a reflection of burnout? Easier to just give benzodiazepine script rather than explore and deal with problems.
- If addicted or under stress may need advice on BMA/LMC counselling services or support group for addicted physicians.

Issues for the practice

- If there are concerns over this doctor's fitness to practise, you should consider reporting them to the GMC.
- If criminal activity is suspected, you may need to involve the police.
- There may be legal implications, eg litigation against the practice for inappropriate prescribing.
- The audit may highlight issues about repeat prescribing policy. Is it computerised, allowing closer monitoring and audit? Are systems in place to prevent excessive repeats?
- Involve local pharmacy advisors to help improve prescribing.
- Consider tackling the problems of the patients on benzodiazepines.
- Consider re-audit after changes have been implemented.

Issues for society

- Minimise prescription fraud – better monitoring and prevention strategies.
- Better services for drug addicts may reduce value of drugs such as benzodiazepines on the streets.
- This problem may eventually be detected by reappraisal/revalidation systems if missed by the practice.

Answer 3

A 40-year-old civil engineer comes to you having been recently diagnosed with retinitis pigmentosa (autosomal dominant). He has two teenage daughters. What factors affect this consultation?

Retinitis pigmentosa is an autosomal dominant condition leading to progressive loss of sight.

Issues for the patient

- Devastating diagnosis. May show bereavement-type reaction – denial, anger, distress.
- No curative treatment available – feeling of powerlessness.
- An independent professional man may find it difficult to ask for help or show vulnerability.
- He may have received limited information at secondary care level. Is he aware of others who have the condition? Does a parent or other family member have condition? What are his ideas, concerns and expectations?
- If no family members are affected there may be a possibility of paternity disputes.

Implications

- Work: May eventually have to give up. Loss of independence/autonomy/income, together with loss of profession, pride in skills, social standing. May need re-training. Possible retirement on disability.
- Family: Guilt/distress over family implications (eg income if cannot work), genetic risks (eg concern about children/future pregnancies). May affect relationship with wife/sex life. Does he have a good support network?

Issues for the doctor

- Potentially a long and difficult consultation which may over-run.

- Need to listen, be sympathetic. Aim to develop good relationship for future, for long-term support.
- Assess needs at this stage – what does he want? Does he need more information on diagnosis?
- Is he seeking testing for daughters or advice on how to break news to family?
- How well do you know this patient? Does he have other medical problems? What are his coping mechanisms?
- Assess for serious psychological distress – depression, suicide risk, drug/alcohol abuse.
- Practical issues: may need period off work to allow to adjust to diagnosis. At some stage he will need to notify his employer and the DVLA. Consider advice from specialist/occupational health.
- Has implications for mortgage/insurance applications.
- Offer contacts eg RNIB, self-help groups, leaflets. Will need specialist input, eg ophthalmology, geneticist.
- Appreciate your own emotions: you may be similar in age, professional with children. Recognise need to offload/discuss with colleague/raise with peers at young principals group.
- Possible area of limited knowledge – may make you uncomfortable.
- Need to address any learning needs for future consultations.

Issues for the teenage daughters

- They may inherit the condition. Frightening diagnosis.
- Are they patients of yours? Decision needed with family on when to inform them. They have a right to know.
- Are they competent to give consent for testing?
- Implications for career choice, driving licence, having a family, life insurance.
- Consider referral to local genetics service who have experience in counselling family members and offering support. Can put them in touch with other affected families.

Issues for the spouse/partner

- When to tell them: may not be ready yet. Respect confidentiality.
- Implications for partner: may have to become breadwinner, potential financial difficulties for family. Psychological impact of diagnosis and prospect of husband's and daughters' disability.
- May have to become a carer.

Wider issues

- Limited provision of geneticists. Increasing recognition of genetic

contribution to disease. Needs more funding.
- Often lack of knowledge in primary care about genetic conditions. Rapidly expanding area of medicine needing better training and dissemination of information to GPs.

Answer 4

PCTs are increasingly looking to explain variation in referral rates to lower secondary care costs. Comment on the literature relating to referral management.

- The unique position of GPs in the NHS – combining the roles of patient advocate and gatekeeper – has raised the possibility of reducing secondary care costs by concentrating on referral rates.
- Referral rates are unsatisfactory indicators of quality because they can hide failures to refer as well as unnecessary referrals.

1 How and why do referrals vary?

Referral rates are reported to vary by three- to four-fold among GPs.

Doctor factors

- GPs who dislike uncertainty or perceive serious disease to be more frequent refer more patients [1].
- Doctors with more experience in an area may be more aware of therapeutic options and refer more.

Patient factors

- A survey of referrals in Nottinghamshire [2] found deprivation accounted for 23% of the variation.

Other factors

- A comparison of referrals between US and UK primary care doctors [3] found 1:7 British patients were referred per annum compared with 1:3 American. This is largely due to long waiting times and low availability of specialists, but also partly due to wider breadth of skills in primary care in the UK.

2 Are referrals avoidable?

- A study of 170 consecutive referrals from one GP [4], reported in the *British Medical Journal* in 1994, concluded that at least one-third potentially avoidable if alternative resources had been available, eg lack of CPNs.

- Large proportion of avoidable referrals are due to insufficient knowledge or experience of the GP.
- Admission rates seem to correlate well with referral rates, implying that referrals are appropriate [5].
- A systematic review in 2000 [1] concluded that GP and patient characteristics explained less than 50% of the variation, and that guidelines had limited effect.

3 How can referral rates be modified?

Feedback

- Feedback of referral rates is ineffective, largely due to scepticism about their quality – that they are a marker of poor quality.

Guidelines

- In March 2002, NICE published referral guidelines for GPs. These have been criticised as being rather simplistic.
- A trial on referral guidelines for infertility in 2001 [6] concluded that these made a small difference in referral practices but no change in outcomes or costs.
- A review in *Family Practice* [1] concluded that rather than targeting high or low referrers through clinical guidelines, activity should concentrate on increasing the number of appropriate referrals, regardless of the referral rate. Pressure on GPs to review their referral behaviour through the use of guidelines may reduce their willingness to tolerate uncertainty and manage problems in primary care, resulting in an increase in referrals to secondary care.

Education

- Educational packages for management of menorrhagia reduced referral rates for hysterectomy, and increased the number of patients treated appropriately with hormonal therapy [7].
- Trials on education of patients suggest that when given evidence-based information regarding surgery for prostatism they are less likely to want referral [8].

Money

- Increasing the provision of minor surgery in primary care under fund-holding uncovered new demand, with minimal effect on secondary care [9].

References

1 Variation in GP referral rates: what can we learn from the literature? [review] *Family Practice* 2000; 17: 462 – 471

2 The effect of deprivation on variations in general practitioners' referral rates: a cross sectional study of computerised data on new medical and surgical outpatient referrals in Nottinghamshire. *British Medical Journal* 1997; 314: 1458 – 1461

3 Comparison of specialty referral rates in the United Kingdom and the United States: retrospective cohort analysis. *British Medical Journal* 2002; 325: 370 – 371

4 Avoidable referrals? Analysis of 170 consecutive referrals to secondary care. *British Medical Journal* 1994; 309: 576 – 578

5 Relation between general practices' outpatient referral rates and rates of elective admission to hospital. *British Medical Journal* 1990; 301: 273 – 276

6 Pragmatic randomised controlled trial to evaluate guidelines for the management of infertility across the primary care-secondary care interface. *British Medical Journal* 2001; 322: 1282 – 1284

7 Randomised controlled trial of educational package on management of menorrhagia in primary care: the Anglia menorrhagia education study. *British Medical Journal* 1999; 318: 1246 – 1250

8 The effect of a shared decision-making program on rates of surgery for benign prostatic hyperplasia. *Medical Care* 1995; 33: 765 – 770

9 Prospective study of trends in referral patterns in fundholding and non-fundholding practices in the Oxford region, 1990 – 4. *British Medical Journal* 1995; 311: 1205 – 1208

Answer 5

How can burnout be avoided?

A recent BMA survey showed the effect of ever-increasing demands on the profession, with more GPs electing to work reduced hours and opting for early retirement. Recognition of burnout and its causes is increasingly important in a career in primary care.

Factors in oneself

• Balance between work and relaxation: engage in outside activities, avoid taking work home, use strategies to 'switch off'.
• Choose a post to best suit your personality and skills, eg size of practice, workload, type of surgery (rural/urban).

- You need to get on with colleagues. Look at options to explore interests, eg hospital posts (clinical assistants), PCT work.
- Consider provision in partnership agreement, eg sabbaticals.
- Look after your own health: Register with GP, avoid self-diagnosis or medication. Exercise regularly. Take care with alcohol/smoking/drug misuse.
- Inability to admit when under stress may exacerbate problems. Be honest with yourself and your partners.

Practical methods

- Find a confidant(e) to share problems, eg difficult patients, complaints, terminally ill patients and practice problems.
- Find mentors from other practices, eg by reciprocal arrangement.
- Keep motivated by engaging in continuing education, try to learn new skills, keep up to date. PLPs may make this more interactive and more enjoyable.
- Young principals groups and/or meeting colleagues provide support, socially and educationally.
- Be aware of resources available if problems develop, eg BMA counselling service, LMC support available, local educational supervisors.

Practice considerations

- Encourage supportive practice environment – hold regular practice meetings and identify problems early.
- Non-critical discussions of practice, eg significant event monitoring.
- Flexibility in practice, eg support outside activities.
- Hold away-days or team building activities for all staff, to encourage cohesiveness. Stress management courses are an option.
- Ensure all are involved in decision making – gives a sense of ownership. Recognise signs of stress early in colleagues – anger, depression, loss of motivation, time off work, signs of alcohol/drug abuse, clinical mistakes, increased complaints.
- Intervene early, eg a meeting to discuss concerns allowing early referral for help/education. Offer options such as reducing hours, less out of hours, time off, less non-clinical work (but impact on other staff may cause resentment).

Local issues

- Deprived or rural areas often have inadequate numbers of GPs, resulting in more work and difficulty recruiting. PMS contracts may help overcome this with salaried posts.

- Single-handed or rural GPs may feel isolated and find difficulty in taking time off or finding a locum.
- Financial support from PCT for practice away-days, eg locum funding may help, especially for small practices. Consider 'locum insurance' to allow sick leave without guilt.
- Provision of good, well-organised and well-staffed out-of-hours service, with option of reducing commitment may help reduce stress, especially with drivers for security.

National strategies

- Government initiatives to reduce work load and improve morale, eg reduction in paperwork, less frequent changes to practice.
- Delegation of clinical work to nurses and non-clinical work to others such as clerical staff.
- Increase GP numbers through increased number of medical students and making general practice more attractive to young doctors. Better remuneration and more respect.
- Encourage culture of openness about mistakes in NHS with stress seen less as a sign of weakness. Mistakes should be admitted without fear of retribution. Care of self should be seen as important part of good practice.
- Better funding available for support services, eg occupational health services for GPs. Easier access to help at all stages of medical career.

Answer 6

Discuss the evidence relating to the following interventions in osteoarthritis:

1   Physiotherapy

- A recent study in the *British Medical Journal*[1] of home exercise for osteoarthritis knee found highly significant reductions in pain at two years. A systematic review in *Bandolier*[2] found small to modest improvements, but pooled osteoarthritis of the hips and knees.
- Knee taping to tilt the patella medially has been shown to reduce knee pain by 25%[3].
- Exercise and weight loss in overweight and obese patients was superior to either intervention in the Arthritis, Diet, and Activity Promotion trial (ADAPT)[4], with significant improvement in activity and knee pain.

2   Steroid injections

- A systematic review in *British Medical Journal*[5] confirmed efficacy of steroid injections for several weeks after injection, although there was an apparently strong placebo response.

3   Dietary supplements

* Evidence [6] suggests fruit and vegetable intake (probably through micronutrients such as magnesium, potassium, etc.) is associated with bone health and markers of bone metabolism.
* Meta-analysis of trials of chondroitin [7] showed it to be effective in reducing pain, improving function and reducing NSAID consumption.
* A Cochrane review of glucosamine [8] confirmed a dose of 1500 mg equivalent in efficacy to ibuprofen and some evidence [9] is there that it may reduce radiographic loss of joint space.

4   Topical and oral anti-inflammatories and analgesics

* A combination of diclofenac with an absorption enhancer was significantly better than placebo in an RCT [10] for pain and stiffness, with efficacy comparable with oral diclofenac.
* A meta-analysis in the *British Medical Journal* in 2004 [11] found that despite initial improvement, after two weeks the effects of topical NSAIDs were similar to placebo.
* The IPSO study [12] compared paracetamol with ibuprofen in osteoarthritis of the hip and knee and found significantly less pain and stiffness in the ibuprofen arm. This confirmed earlier reports [13] that paracetamol had no significant effect in osteoarthritis of the knee.

References

1   Home based exercise programme for knee pain and knee osteoarthritis: randomised controlled clinical trial. *British Medical Journal* 2002; 325: 752

2   Osteoarthritis of the knee: keep it taped. *Bandolier* (www.jr2.ox.ac.uk/bandolier)

3   Effectiveness of exercise therapy in patients with osteoarthritis of the hip or knee. *Arthritis and Rheumatism* 1999; 42: 1361–1369

4   Exercise and dietary weight loss in overweight and obese older adults with knee osteoarthritis: the arthritis, diet, and activity promotion trial. *Arthritis and Rheumatism* 2004; 50: 1501–1510

5   Corticosteroid injections for osteoarthritis of the knee: meta-analysis. *British Medical Journal* 2004; 328: 869–870

6   Dietary influences on bone mass and bone metabolism: further evidence of a positive link between fruit and vegetable consumption and bone health. *American Journal of Clinical*

Nutrition 2000: 71; 142 – 151
7 A meta-analysis of chondroitin sulphate in the treatment of
osteoarthritis. *J Rheumatology* 2000;27:205 – 211
8 'Glucosamine therapy for treating osteoarthritis.' The Cochrane
Database of systematic reviews 2000, Issue 2. Art. No.:
CD002946. DOI: 10.1002/14651858.CD0022946
9 Long term effects of glucosamine sulphate on osteoarthritis
progression: a randomised controlled clinical trial. *The Lancet*
2001; 357: 251
10 Efficacy and safety of a topical diclofenac solution (Pennsaid) in
the treatment of primary osteoarthritis of the knee: a randomised,
double blind, vehicle controlled clinical trial. *Archives of Internal
Medicine* 2004; 164: 2017 – 2023
11 Efficacy of topical NSAIDs in the treatment of osteoarthritis:
meta-analysis of randomised controlled trials. *British Medical
Journal* 2004; 329: 324
12 The IPSO study: ibuprofen, paracetamol study in osteoarthritis.
Annals of the Rheumatic Diseases 2004; 63: 1028 – 1034
13 Paracetamol in osteoarthritis of the knee. *Annals of the Rheumatic
Diseases* 2004; 63: 923 – 930

Answer 7

**As a result of an audit it has become clear that an excessive
number of your patients fail to attend outpatient appointments
after being referred by their GP. In a drive to improve access
times you set up a working party to explore the causes of this.
You wish the process to be evidence based.**

1 **Outline how you would gather the evidence**

- Define a question, eg 'Why do patients fail to attend their
appointments?'
- Identify and search resource areas:
  - Medline for worldwide literature search. Needs precise searching
methodology. Local medical librarian may be of help.
  - Internet search of *British Medical Journal* archive, again with
clearly defined search terms and knowledge of system. Could
also try Royal College of General Practitioners website for
references to back issues of *British Journal of General Practice*.
  - Textbooks. Local medical library may have access to useful
textbooks, eg *Notes for the MRCGP*, which summarise research
findings in some areas.
  - Word of mouth. Talking over with colleagues may open lines of
inquiry. Potentially rewarding, but also potentially misleading.

- Agree screening process, eg priority for recent publications in respected peer reviewed journals (eg *British Medical Journal, British Journal of General Practice*) that are directly relevant. Consider hierarchy of evidence, with RCTs at the top and case reports at the bottom.
- Need to distinguish between qualitative and quantitative evidence. For an area like this there is likely to be plenty of qualitative evidence regarding causes and possibly quantitative evidence regarding possible solutions. For qualitative data the RCT is the gold standard, for qualitative data this is seldom practical.
- Screen results, selecting the most relevant that satisfy the above criteria.
- Summarise relevant data.

2   **Read reference material 7.1a, part of a paper from the *British Journal of General Practice* entitled 'Patient, hospital and general practitioner characteristics associated with non-attendance: a cohort study' (with copyright permission from the *British Journal of General Practice* 2002; 52: 317–319). Comment on the strengths and weaknesses of the methodology of the study as presented**

Strengths

- Journal: peer reviewed journal, relevant to UK general practice.
- Study design: systematic approach studying all GP referrals avoids inclusion bias.
- Study population: Jarman score calculated from postcode, giving a quantifiable estimate of deprivation.
- Statistical analysis: validated method of comparing populations. Clearly defined variables.
- All patients accounted for in data.

Weaknesses

- Study design: prospective cohort study, potential for bias as GPs may be aware they are being studied and stress importance of attendance or alter referring habits. Running in parallel with an RCT will limit study design; unclear if this was on same patients, in which case potential bias from intervention.
- Studied all referrals from 26 GPs in 13 practices. Why so few GPs? Did some of the GPs in these practices object (source of possible inclusion bias)? How were they selected?
- Study population: patients in Exeter may not be representative of patients in the rest of the UK, eg socio-economic and ethnic

differences. This may limit applicability of study. Need baseline data on these variables. Referral rates calculated from referrals during study, may not be representative either because of GPs knowing they are being observed or seasonal variation, particularly as the study only looked at data from January to May.

Answer 8

1   Extracts from the results section of the paper referred to in the Question 7 are given in reference material 7.2a (with copyright permission from the *British Journal of General Practice*). What do you conclude from the results presented?

Characteristics of non-attenders compared with attenders and cancellations

- The mean age, sex and interval between referral and appointment are all statistically significant as analysed in these results, with p values < 0.05.
- The confidence interval for sex distribution in the non-attenders is wide. A larger cohort may reduce the percentage of males closer to that of the attender group, which has narrower confidence intervals owing to its large size.
- The mean ages are markedly different with relatively narrow confidence intervals, suggesting this is a real difference, combined with a p value < 0.0001.
- The multivariable analysis of characteristics of non-attendance suggest that male sex, age, Jarman score and interval to appointment are all statistically significant, with p values < 0.05.

Characteristics of GPs

- The median interval between referral and appointment similarly has a statistically significant p value of < 0.0001 but the confidence intervals are wide. A larger cohort would probably reduce this.
- The percentages for GPs by fundholding and MRCGP status are not significant, both with p values > 0.05. The referral rate is borderline, with a p value of 0.05.

2   What other factors may explain the results seen?

There are several possible areas of confounding:

- The non-attender cohort is relatively small, increasing the chance of misleading results.
- The conditions for which the non-attenders were referred may have

been self-limiting, eg rashes.
- Some of the non-attenders may have been treated with an acute presentation of their problem while waiting. Similarly they may have moved away from the area, died or had the operation carried out privately.
- Knowing the breakdown by specialty might provide more useful data, as all of the non-attenders may be clustered in one specialty with a particularly long waiting list skewing the average results.
- Geographical distance from hospital and transport options may also provide bias. Patients with their own transport are more likely to attend.
- Did the patients who failed to attend receive their appointment letters? Is there a problem with up-to-date records of addresses? Areas with high Jarman scores often have a high proportion of rented accommodation and itinerant populations.
- Another possibility is that the specialists or GPs may be giving preferential treatment to certain groups of patients with earlier appointments.

Answer 9

1   **How does the literature contribute to the diagnosis and initial assessment of chronic obstructive pulmonary disease (COPD)?**

- NICE guidelines [1] suggest diagnosis should be considered in patients over the age of 35 years who have a risk factor (generally smoking) and who present with exertional breathlessness, chronic cough, regular sputum production, frequent winter 'bronchitis' or wheeze. The presence of airflow obstruction should be confirmed by spirometry. These patients do not require reversibility testing, although this may be useful to exclude asthma [2].
- Look for complications, eg cor pulmonale, and identify those in need of specialist referral.
- Initial assessment should include screening for depression, which is common and recording BMI with nutritional supplements if low.
- The guidelines also stress importance of measuring health status rather than relying on FEV_1 as a guide to disease progression.
- The nGMS quality and outcomes framework does, however, require spirometry including reversibility testing and recording of FEV_1 every 27 months.

2   Describe the step-wise use of initial therapy for COPD with an
     algorithm

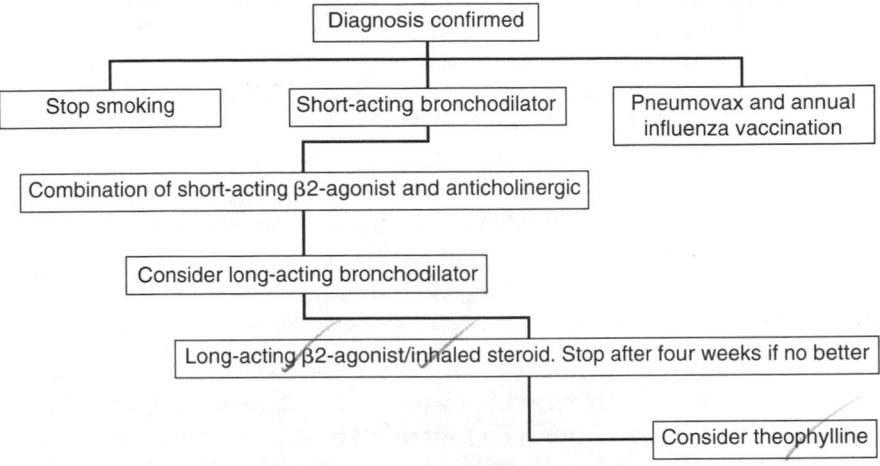

3   How does the literature contribute to the management of
     exacerbations of COPD?

- NICE guidelines suggest treating exacerbations with increased
  frequency of bronchodilator use – consider giving via a nebuliser,
  oral antibiotics if purulent sputum, prednisolone 30 mg daily for
  7–14 days – for all patients with significant increase in
  breathlessness, and all patients admitted to hospital, unless
  contraindicated.
- Where purulent cough is a problem, consider use of
  N-acetylcysteine.
- The NICE guidelines recommend the use of self-management plans
  with a supply of steroids and antibiotics to use early in
  exacerbations.
- Evidence suggests that hospital-at-home schemes may be useful in
  managing exacerbations of COPD [3], with similar outcomes and
  substantially reduced costs.
- Community-based pulmonary rehabilitation [4] after admission to
  hospital for acute exacerbations of COPD is safe and leads to
  statistically and clinically significant improvements in exercise
  capacity and health status at three months.

References

1 NICE clinical guideline 12.2004. (www.nice.org.uk)
2 Guidelines for chronic obstructive pulmonary disease.*British Medical Journal* 2004; 329: 363–364
3 Hospital at home for patients with acute exacerbations of chronic obstructive pulmonary disease: systematic review of evidence. *British Medical Journal* 2004; 329: 315
4 Community pulmonary rehabilitation after hospitalisation for acute exacerbations of chronic obstructive pulmonary disease: randomised controlled study. *British Medical Journal* November 2004; 329: 1209

Answer 10

While looking at ways to improve the care of patients with epilepsy in your practice, you come across the paper 'A pragmatic randomised controlled trial of a prompt and reminder card in the care of people with epilepsy' (with permission from the *British Journal of General Practice* 2002; 52: 93–98; reference material 7.3a).

1 Comment on the strengths and weaknesses of the method described

Strengths

- The study is general practice based, making it relevant to primary care management.
- The search criteria for identifying patients through a summary and medication search are appropriate to identify suitable patients.
- Practice selection was at random in the four areas, reducing the likelihood of inclusion bias.
- The intervention was a simple, standardised evidence-based prompt. This was designed to be easy to use in conjunction with medical records.
- Outcome measures were objective, allowing direct comparison, eg of seizure frequency.

Weaknesses

- Randomisation was done with a random number table. It is not clear how this was done and whether the stratification of practices before randomisation gave truly equivalent groups. Data on comparison between the three groups were not given.
- Excluding those with learning disabilities makes the results less applicable to these patients, which is unfortunate since they may be

the patients whose care is least satisfactory.
- The doctor-held paper prompt might be less useful in paperless practices where the GPs do not routinely use paper notes.
- The length of the paper prompt might act as a disincentive during consultations when time is limited.
- The secondary outcomes of retrieval and completion rate of the card are not directly linked to improved quality of care, which was the aim of the trial.

2   **Comment on the results of the trial (shown in Tables 1, 2 and 3 of reference material 7.3b)**

- The data in Table 1 demonstrate that recording of seizure frequency in the notes is poor prior to the intervention, with only 37% of records including these data.
- After the intervention year the recording in the doctor-held record group had improved significantly (odds ratio 1.82, p = 0.003), but not the patient-held group.
- The self-reported seizure frequency data showed an increase in the numbers of patients in all three groups who were seizure free at the end of the intervention, but the increases were not statistically significant.
- The only statistically significant changes in Table 3 are that significantly more patients reported side-effects in the intervention groups and that fewer patients reported satisfaction with GP information provision in the intervention groups.
- There were no differences in pharmacological management.

3   **Comment on possible reasons for these results**

- The increased recording by doctors may be explained by the Hawthorne effect, ie GPs who know they are being watched may concentrate more on data recording.
- These data suggest that the intervention increased recording at the expense of patient satisfaction, ie GPs may have been spending more time filling in record cards rather than listening to their patients. The aim of the intervention should be to improve care, not just to improve record keeping.

Answer 11

Discuss the impact of deprivation on general practice.

Since Tudor Hart described the inverse care law many people have attempted to quantify the effect of deprivation on general practice. The most widely used tools are the Jarman and Townsend indices which use factors such as unemployment, single-parent families and overcrowding.

Social factors

- Higher unemployment, and if employed more likely to work shifts, with longer hours and less holiday and sick pay. May have less disposable income for prescriptions, heating, etc.
- Housing: less likely to have central heating and inside toilets. More likely to be rented accommodation. More likely to be in industrial areas with more pollution. Many rural areas may also be deprived. May be in areas of high crime.
- Access: more reliance on public transport or lifts from friends/family may result in more requests for home visits.
- Social stressors may result in more mental health problems, and certain underprivileged groups more likely in deprived areas, eg asylum seekers, ethnic minorities.
- Drug abuse more common.

Doctor factors

- Demand is higher. More single mothers and people on low incomes.
- More 'difficult' problems, eg drugs, alcohol, psychological problems.
- Communication may be a problem where patients from ethnic minorities may not speak English.
- Security may be an issue, eg an escort may be needed when making home visits in areas of high crime.
- Burnout may be a problem in the face of seemingly insurmountable social problems, with high demand and low resources.

Patient factors

- Higher morbidity and mortality at all ages. Accidents, especially in children, more common. Smoking more common, leading to lower life expectancy due to smoking-related disease, cancers, COPD, cardiovascular disease.
- Less access to preventive services.
- Lifestyle: diet may be poor. Less access to sports facilities, and healthy lifestyle often a low priority.
- Education and literacy: patient leaflets may not be understood, especially among ethnic minorities. Psychiatric morbidity is higher and may be unrecognised.
- Domestic violence and abuse more common.
- In areas of ethnic minorities, uncommon diseases may be seen, eg vitamin D deficient rickets, tuberculosis.
- Households less likely to have telephones, so there may be problems phoning for appointments.

Practice factors

- May have lower income due to poor uptake of immunisations, smears, etc.
- Mobile population, require regular updating of records.
- Need good co-ordination with social services and health visitors.
- Recruitment and retention: vacant posts impact on existing staff. Locums may be hard to find. PMS may help to address this with salaried posts and moving away from traditional incentive payments (eg smears) into more appropriate areas of need (eg drugs, asylum seekers).
- Practice leaflets need to be appropriate for patients' language and literacy levels.
- Appointments: approximately 50% higher consultation rate. Chronic sickness rate is 40% higher in deprived areas. Walk-in surgeries or telephone triage may be more appropriate than traditional systems.
- Vandalism of premises may affect services. Crime including theft of prescription pads and burglary common. Will need good security systems in place and policies for dangerous or difficult patients.
- Health promotion clinics may require novel approaches to increase attendance.
- Interpreters may be required, or staff with language skills.
- Take educational abilities, eg literacy into account when sending letters.

Wider issues

- Holidays/study leave: may be hard to get locums to cover leave, affecting postgraduate education.
- PCT may need to employ locums to fill vacancies or cover holiday or leave.
- PCT may need novel approaches to managing demand, eg PMS contracts, health promotion clinics, walk-in centres etc.
- Some studies suggest bias in waiting times for secondary care services against deprived patients.

Answer 12

A 21-year-old girl and her boyfriend come to you for the morning-after pill. They both have Down's syndrome and attend a local daycare centre. What issues does this raise, and how would you proceed?

This situation poses a number of potential problems. The following points should be borne in mind.

Consultation issues

- Use appropriate language. Assume they are mentally competent unless there is evidence otherwise.
- Beware of conscious or subconscious prejudice.
- Do not assume she waives her confidentiality by bringing boyfriend in.

Ethical issues

- Is she competent?
- Is she at risk?
- Has she fully consented to sex?

Doctor/practice issues

- Does this reflect failure of contraceptive advice?
- Are other areas of sexual health being neglected, eg cervical smears, STD counselling?
- Has she not consulted before because she is always escorted by her parents?
- Has she been put off by previous experience of doctor's attitude, eg patronising attitude?
- Is there a problem with access to healthcare for patients with learning difficulties?

Medical issues

- Is there any medical condition that makes pregnancy dangerous (eg congenital heart disease) or puts her at risk of venous thromboembolism?
- Could she be pregnant from earlier incidents?

Legal issues

- Meticulous note keeping.
- If not competent, consider contacting defence organisation for advice trying to delay in providing emergency contraception.
- Be prepared for possible problems with parents.

Genetic issues

High risk of offspring with Down's syndrome. Can they understand genetic risk? Respect their opinions.

Management of the problem

- Take a full sexual history: LMP (last menstrual period), dates of unprotected sexual intercourse, usual cycle. Using any contraception?
- Review previous medical history.
- Conduct a brief examination, eg CVS and BP.
- Consider need for pregnancy test if earlier exposures.

Immediate treatment

- If no contraindications and treatment indicated, prescribe emergency contraception or consider emergency coil fitting.
- If not suitable for emergency contraception, seek advice from family planning clinic.
- Check her understanding throughout.
- Ensure she understands possible treatment failure.
- Plan follow-up, in particular future contraception, consider review for pregnancy test.

Future treatment

- Need for effective contraception.
- Consider addressing other sexual health needs, eg smears?

Other issues

- Assess provision of healthcare for patients with learning difficulties.
- If possibility of non-consensual sex, is there a lack of supervision at daycare centre or at home?
- Are practice staff aware of confidentiality/consent issues?

Paper 8

Answer 1

> Hannah, a normally fit and active 3-year-old, is brought to you by her parents. She is lethargic, dehydrated and smells ketotic. A fingerprick BM shows a blood glucose of 22. What are your aims, now and in the future?

You need to be sympathetic to the parents, address their concerns and possible feelings of guilt. Try not to alarm or scare Hannah; talk to and examine her sensitively to put her at ease.

Immediate management

Hannah almost certainly has diabetes. Immediate priorities are:

- Review history: urinary frequency, appetite, weight loss, recent illness.
- Examination: assess respiratory rate, signs of acidosis, dehydration.
- Management: refer immediately to on-call paediatrician for rehydration, confirmation of diagnosis and insulin treatment.
- Explain likely diagnosis and need for investigation and initial treatment in hospital. Offer to telephone later to clarify any queries.

Short-term management

Hannah and her family will need help and support, physically, financially and emotionally.

- Offer advice about support services, eg the British Diabetic Association.
- Look out for guilt in parents, fear of diabetes in siblings and grief reactions as they realise Hannah has lost her excellent health. Look for denial and depression.
- Be aware of possible honeymoon period of low insulin requirements; family may challenge diagnosis.
- Initially most of care will be undertaken by the paediatricians but be prepared to share care later.
- Practice staff, eg health visitor and nurses, may need input to support family.

Long-term management

- Aim for normal quality of life with minimal side-effects and complications.
- Explain that good control may be at the expense of hypos. Prepare them for this if it has not been done so in hospital (DCCT trial).
- Be aware of difficult times, eg exercise, illness, alcohol, school trips, adolescence, etc.
- Ensure nursery/school is happy and confident with care, possibly health visitor to visit.
- Ensure Hannah is on the practice register. Importance of regular follow-up, eg retinal screening, kidney function.
- When she considers planning a family, ensure preconception counselling and consultant-led care.
- Advise on career implications, eg she cannot be a heavy goods vehicle (HGV) driver.

Answer 2

'Growing old gracefully' – how can general practice meet the needs of elderly people?

- The percentage of people aged over 60 years in the UK is predicted to rise from 20% to 30% by 2031.
- The NSF for the Elderly aims to improve health and social care for these individuals with varied physical, practical and emotional needs.

Provision of medical care

- Age should not prejudice provision of treatment. Elderly people often have most to gain from preventive measures, eg anticoagulation in AF to reduce stroke.
- Healthcare advice, eg on weight, smoking, exercise, is never too late and often well received.
- Addressing mental health problems is important. Elderly people have a high incidence of depression, and suicide risk is underestimated. Bereavement may increase depression and social isolation. Need to actively seek mood disturbance and instigate appropriate treatment with minimum side-effects (eg SSRIs), and have access to CPNs to support.
- Elder abuse is not uncommon, and the possibility must be considered.
- Ensure regular review – new targets to achieve over-75 checks.
- May need to actively call patients for review, eg by letter. If unable

to attend, consider home visit by doctor, district nurse or health visitor.
• Appropriate use of medication: physiological changes with ageing may influence side-effects or doses.
• Avoid polypharmacy where possible. Regularly review need for medication, compliance and side-effects. Drugs (eg benzodiazepines) may cause falls or accidents. Ensure that your practice has mechanisms to review repeat prescriptions.
• Ensure relationships are maintained with residential/nursing homes with access to help when needed. Potential benefits of educating staff, eg skin care, prevention of pressure sores, diabetic management.

Accessibility of healthcare

• Consider transport or disabilities affecting ability to attend surgeries. Consider provision of transport, eg for diabetic reviews, etc.
• Involve primary healthcare team, eg health visitor, for home and local daycare visits.
• Provide information on services: surgery contact numbers, NHS Direct, social services, elderly organisations, eg Help the Aged.
• Communication difficulties: facilities for those with visual impairments (eg large print practice leaflet, etc.) and hearing problems (eg induction loops).
• Provision for physical disability, eg hand rails/ramps/lift at entrance. Comfortable spacious waiting area with minimum hazards and possibly raised chairs. Staff should be sensitive to patients who may need assistance.

Addressing non-medical issues

• Aim to reduce social isolation in those living alone with distant relatives unable to provide support. Practice staff need to provide information on resources, eg community buses for shopping, social/luncheon groups, daycare centres.
• Safety at home: ensure provision of aids, eg walking frames, hand rails, home help for cleaning/bathing assistance. Aim to maintain independent living in own home.
• Financial issues: health visitors can help to complete benefit claims, etc.
• Respect autonomy: Competent elderly people have right to refuse help, others may need help (eg in dementia).
• Support for carers is often neglected. Their role can be stressful and isolating. Ensure practice has record of carers. Consider carer support groups, be alert for signs of psychological distress.

- Ensure up-to-date records for elderly patients include next of kin, power of attorney and advance directives.

Implications of improved care

- Workload: good care of elderly people with long complicated consultations, regular reviews and home visits are time consuming for the whole PHCT.
- Financial impact: costs of adaptations to surgery premises, providing transport, and staff time. Ultimately these may be offset by more cost-effective and appropriate prescribing and reduced morbidity from falls, etc.
- Improved patient satisfaction: patients should feel their needs are being addressed, their health is being taken seriously and their independence is being maintained.
- Will need regular audit to ensure aims are being achieved.
- Government requirements to implement the NSF have raised concerns that this represents more work for GPs to reduce hospital admissions. GPs may be required to provide 'intermediate/home care' which increases workload and may not be effective or evidence based. GPs may not have necessary skills.
- Needs considerable extra resources as demand will continue to increase as population grows.

Answer 3

The NSF for Elderly People and Stroke places new emphasis on the prevention and treatment of stroke. See reference material 6.1a, an extract from the paper 'Use of ramipril in preventing stroke: double blind randomised trial' (with permission from *British Medical Journal* 2002; 324: 699).

1   Comment on the methodology of the trial

- The study was a randomised double blind controlled trial. This is the gold standard study design.
- The study addressed a well-formulated question: Does ramipril prevent stroke in high risk patients? The study design was appropriate to answer this.
- The population was selected to be high risk for stroke. The exclusion criteria were reasonable and did not exclude too many patient groups.
- The intervention was similar to the standard use of ramipril in everyday practice, with monitoring of renal function, and the patients received no other intervention.
- All patients were put on the maximal ramipril dose. In practice this

may not be tolerated by many patients. Data on the effectiveness of lower doses are not available, so the results may not be representative for patients on lower doses.
- Baseline characteristics are given but not split into intervention and control. Method of recruitment and randomisation are not given, although a reference is made to earlier publications.
- Follow-up was excellent with 99.9% follow-up achieved.
- The outcomes were clinically appropriate endpoints of myocardial infarction, stroke or cardiovascular death. Stroke was diagnosed by CT where possible and an adjudication committee decided on diagnoses using records. Recovery was judged according to a standardised six-point scale, reducing recall and observer bias.

2   **Comment on the results in Table 1 of reference material 8.1b**

- The results show a reduction in total strokes from 4.9% to 3.4%, a relative risk (RR) reduction of 32%.
- The reductions here are 1.0 % to 0.4% (RR reduction 61%) for fatal strokes and 3.9% to 3.0% (RR reduction 24%) for non-fatal strokes.
- The reductions are seen in both ischaemic and non-ischaemic strokes.
- The table does not give p values, but the confidence intervals for all of these are consistent with a positive effect except for non-ischaemic stroke where the confidence intervals cross 1.
- These results appear to support the hypothesis that ramipril reduces the incidence of stroke.

3   **Comment on the statement from the conclusion 'Widespread use of an angiotensin converting enzyme inhibitor such as ramipril in patients at high risk of stroke is likely to have a major impact on public health'**

- The results of this study, while showing impressive relative risk reductions are less impressive when absolute risk reductions are considered.
  - For total strokes the ARR is 1.5%, ie a number needed to treat (NNT) of 67 to prevent 1 stroke.
  - For non-fatal strokes the ARR is 0.9%, ie an NNT of 111 to prevent 1 non-fatal stroke.
  - For fatal strokes the ARR is 0.6%, ie an NNT of 166 to prevent 1 fatal stroke.
- The side-effects of ramipril are not insignificant, with a small number developing worsening renal impairment as a result.
- The funds necessary to implement the prescribing of ramipril in all patients at high risk might be better spent in funding rehabilitation services.

Answer 4

The practice receptionist points out that there seem to be a large number of patients not attending appointments. What do you need to consider when looking at this problem?

- Patients missing appointments waste a considerable amount of resources and contribute to long access times.
- The first step is to assess the scale of the problem by auditing non-attenders. Involve receptionists, eg record over a 1-month period. Determine acceptable levels given the practice demographics (eg level of deprivation).
- Which groups of patients appear to miss appointments?
- Do the numbers vary between different partners or with locums?

What issues need to be considered with regard to DNA rates?

Patient issues

- May be legitimate reasons for not attending – family/work crisis, car breakdown, no access to telephone.
- Misinterpretation of time when booking, eg not written down, forgotten.
- Limited access early in illness may lead to recovery or seeking help elsewhere, eg A&E or walk-in centre.
- Patients with sensitive or embarrassing problems may lose courage to attend or be put off by questioning from receptionists.
- Fail to realise importance of cancelling to free-up spaces.
- Some patients are embarrassed to cancel – easier just not to turn up.
- Some patients are just unreliable.

Doctor issues

- You may welcome a few non-attenders. The space provides an opportunity to catch up if running behind, make phone calls and have a coffee.
- You may feel angry about the waste of time and lack of courtesy to cancel.
- High non-attendance rates increase waiting times, affecting other patients.
- For important consultations, eg to discuss abnormal test results, chasing patients by phone or letter is more time consuming and frustrating.
- Non-attendance may be related to your consulting style, unnecessary follow-ups, or poor communication with patients.
- You may habitually run late, causing patient frustration.

Practice nurse/physiotherapist issues

- Issues similar to doctors. Appointments often longer, even more time wasted.
- Patients may see nurse appointments as second best and fail to attend.

Reducing numbers

- Patient questionnaires may explore cause and suggest strategies to reduce missed appointments.
- Posters highlighting importance of cancelling appointments if patient can not attend. Clearly state in practice leaflet.
- Particular groups or families who frequently fail to attend may be identified and reminded, but this is time consuming.
- Consider warning or removal from list for patients who frequently fail to attend.
- Issue written confirmation of appointment time when booking.
- Improve access – aim for 24/48 h, look at Advanced Access strategies.
- Review follow-up appointments. Are they all necessary? Pass responsibility to patient to re-attend if not improving.
- Increase appointment time to, eg, 15 minutes – may improve patient satisfaction and reduce re-attendance.
- Re-audit after changes implemented.

Local issues

- Do local practices have similar problems? Are more GPs needed?
- Is access in tune to local needs? Offer variety of sources to access medical help at convenient times, eg walk-in centre, more nurse-led minor illness clinics. May need targeted funding.
- Danger that easier access may increase demand.
- Non-attendance in primary care may be mirrored in secondary care, affecting access here.
- Consider community media campaign highlighting impact of non-attendance on resources for NHS and waiting lists.

Answer 5

A 30-year-old woman with a BMI of 32 comes to see you requesting a prescription for slimming drugs which she read about in a magazine. What issues does this consultation raise?

Obesity is a major health problem in developed countries, increasing the risk of conditions such as diabetes mellitus, ischaemic heart disease and joint disease. These patients are a significant drain on health service resources.

Issues raised by this consultation

Patient issues

- Why has she presented now? Does she or a family member have an obesity-related illness? Is she experiencing relationship or work problems? Is she happy with her weight but has been encouraged to attend by a partner, relative or boss?
- Does she have poor self-esteem or psychological illness, eg depression? Is she being victimised about her weight?
- Any hidden agendas, eg concern about polycystic ovaries or infertility?
- What are her ideas about weight loss and diet? Has she tried other diets or slimming clubs?
- Does she have friends who have tried medications? Are her expectations realistic?

Doctor issues

- Sensitive issue. Importance of rapport. Be non-judgemental with regular follow-up.
- Exclude secondary causes (eg hypothyroidism, Cushing's) and co-morbidity (eg BP, diabetes).
- Question about other risk factors, eg smoking, alcohol. Is she on the pill? Obesity is a relative contraindication.
- Aim to explore her understanding of obesity and its risks. What interventions has she tried before? May benefit from referral to dietician.
- If considering medication explain that she needs to achieve initial weight loss with diet alone, exclude contraindications, counsel about side-effects, monitoring and length of treatment.
- Potentially a long and stressful consultation with implications for time management.
- Any learning needs regarding obesity management and drug treatments?
- Need to be aware of NICE guidance on prescribing criteria for orlistat and sibutramine.
- Doctor prejudices may affect consultation, eg see obesity as lack of self-control and the patient's own responsibility rather than a medical issue.

Practice issues

- Increasingly common reason for consultation – often long, frequent appointments which use a lot of GP time.
- Often involve practice nurses for weight monitoring and dietary advice. Nurses need education on obesity management.
- Resources should be available in the practice for patients, eg leaflets, diet sheets and videos.
- Consider setting up a patient support group, but may have time and resource implications.
- If this is an area of interest for partner or nurse consider establishing dedicated obesity clinic.

Wider issues

- Are anti-obesity drugs expensive 'lifestyle drugs' which burden the cash limited NHS?
- Obesity is a major health problem, using valuable NHS resources.
- Should PCTs fund community dieticians, community-led support groups, subsidy for membership of gyms, etc.?
- Controversies over efficacy and safety, eg concerns about NICE guidance.
- Issues regarding society's attitude to weight in general, the media portrayal of thinness as ideal.
- Should we lobby government and the food industry to improve quality and pricing of foods?
- Aim to educate children and improve quality of school meals, and make exercise attractive, accessible and affordable.

Answer 6

Discuss the available evidence regarding screening and prevention of type 2 diabetes.

Prevention

- An editorial in the *British Medical Journal* in 2002[1] argued that we should attempt to target pre-diabetes.
- Data from trials have shown that lifestyle interventions (weight loss and exercise) reduce the incidence of diabetes 59%[2] with an NNT of 6.9 over three years' treatment.
- Another editorial has argued that controlling obesity in the UK is critical not only in prevention of type 2 diabetes but also in its treatment[3]. It also points out that a substantially increased awareness of risk factors such as obesity and impaired glucose

tolerance is needed among doctors.

- A bigger obstacle still is that lifestyle and body weight are far from being under voluntary control, and so prevention of diabetes requires sustained cultural change.
- The Nurses' Health Study [4] showed that the risk of diabetes in women with a BMI of 29–31 was 28 times higher than those with a BMI of 22, while for those with a BMI over 35 the risk was 93 times higher. This prospective study of 84 941 female nurses followed for 16 years also found a combination of five modifiable risk factors related to dietary behaviour, physical activity, weight, and cigarette smoking was identified that was associated with a remarkable 91% reduction in the risk of developing diabetes. Even with a family history of diabetes the risk reduction was 88% [5].
- In the Finnish diabetes prevention study weight loss in overweight subjects with impaired glucose tolerance, averaging just 3–4 kg over four years, led to a 58% reduction in incident diabetes [6].
- South Asians are at increased risk of diabetes and its complications. An editorial in the *British Medical Journal* in 2003 [7] suggested adopting a lower level of BMI of 23 as overweight in South Asians, and also stated that the particular educational needs of South Asian communities need to be addressed.
- Knowledge of the risks of increasing obesity is poor among these communities, and culturally appropriate interventions are required that involve a whole community, eg 'Project Dil' in Leicester [8], where focus groups identified the South Asian communities' needs, engaged primary care to set up training programmes for patients and healthcare professionals, and developed peer educators to spread the message.
- Healthcare professionals need to understand better the higher risks of coronary heart disease and diabetes and lower thresholds for intervention required in South Asian people.
- Compared with European patients, lower thresholds for intervention with regard to high BP, dyslipidaemias, or glycaemia should be considered in South Asian patients with diabetes because of their higher risk for complications.

Screening

- The NSF for Diabetes states that 'The NHS will develop, implement and monitor strategies to identify people who do not know that they have diabetes'. The arguments for screening are:
  - diabetes is common
  - it is an important public health problem
  - many patients have complications at diagnosis

- reliable treatment exists and will affect disease prognosis if instituted early (UKPDS, DCCT), ie it fulfils many of Wilson and Junger's criteria.
- One proposed screening strategy is to screen everyone over the age of 45 years with a triennial fasting blood glucose (American Diabetes Association). Arguments against this are that it would be time consuming, expensive in terms of manpower and will screen the worried-well rather than high-risk groups.
- An alternative suggestion is to target those at risk, eg those who are obese or have hypertension or a strong family history. A trial of universal screening in primary care detected positive results in 0.2% of those with no risk factors, but 2.8% in high-risk groups [9].
- A primary care-based study reported in *Bandolier* [10] suggested that undiagnosed diabetes rates of 20% of those already diagnosed, and that screening by age and BMI, was an effective tool with numbers needed to test of 7 for BMI over 30 and age >65 years.

References

1 Targeting people with pre-diabetes [editorial]. *British Medical Journal* 2002; 325: 403 – 404
2 Diabetes Prevention Program Research Group. Reduction in the incidence of type 2 diabetes with lifestyle intervention or metformin. *New England Journal of Medicine* 2002; 346: 393 – 403
3 Prevention and cure of type 2 diabetes [editorial]. *British Medical Journal* 2002; 325: 232 – 233
4 Weight as a risk factor for clinical diabetes in women. *American Journal of Epidemiology* 1990; 132: 501 – 513
5 Diet, lifestyle, and the risk of type 2 diabetes mellitus in women. *New England Journal of Medicine* 2001; 345: 790 – 797
6 Prevention of Type 2 diabetes mellitus by changes in lifestyle among subjects with impaired glucose tolerance, *New England Journal of Medicine* 2001; 344: 1343 – 1350.
7 Preventing Diabetes in South Asians [editorial]. *British Medical Journal* 2003; 327: 1059 – 1060
8 Project Dil: a co-ordinated primary care and community health promotion programme for reducing risk factors of coronary heart disease amongst the South Asian community in Leicester – experiences and evaluation of the project. *Ethnic Health* 2001; 6: 265 – 70
9 Screening for diabetes in general practice: cross sectional population study. *British Medical Journal* 2001; 323: 548
10 A simple pragmatic system for detecting new cases of type 2

diabetes and impaired fasting glycaemia in primary care. *Family Practice* 2004: 21; 57 – 62

Answer 7

Comment on the evidence relating to the management of hay fever.

General allergen avoidance measures

- This has been discussed in a *British Journal of General Practice* editorial [1]. Includes avoiding picnics, camping and cutting grass, wearing wraparound sunglasses when outdoors, washing hair and showering on return from countryside, washing pets regularly, holidaying by seaside and mountainous areas rather than farms, closing bedroom windows and keeping car windows up when driving.
- Individuals may have some clues as to their specific sensitivity which may help avoid symptoms, eg symptoms in April suggests tree pollens whereas symptoms in May suggests grass pollen. Fungal spores cause problems through to September.

Treatment of symptoms

- A *MeReC Bulletin* [2] suggests treatment choice is a balance between symptom pattern and patient preference.
- Intranasal corticosteroids are the treatment of choice in patients with moderate to severe symptoms as they relieve all symptoms. Must be used regularly to be effective and maximum efficacy develops over several weeks. Start two weeks before symptoms due.
- Oral antihistamines are effective for ocular symptoms, rhinorrhoea and sneezing but do not affect congestion. More rapid onset of action than nasal steroids and can be taken prn.
- No significant difference has been found between second-generation (eg loratadine) and third-generation (eg desloratadine) oral antihistamines in terms of efficacy.
- Topical antihistamines have more rapid onset (15 minutes vs 1 – 3 hours) but do not affect congestion.
- If maximal medication is not controlling symptoms, check compliance in particular with nasal spray use.
- If compliance is good and there are special circumstances, eg exams consider a short course of oral steroids.
- Depot steroids are more likely to cause adrenal suppression and are not now considered a suitable treatment for hay fever.

Immunotherapy

- Allergen-specific immunotherapy may be effective in desensitisation of patients with allergic rhinitis, but risk of life-threatening anaphylaxis, especially in a group at risk of severe allergic reaction, resulted in the Committee on Safety of Medicines concluding that it should not be used.

Alternative therapies

- Evidence from randomised controlled trials suggest butterbur may be as effective as cetirizine in reducing symptoms, although no placebo was used and some preparations of butterbur are potentially toxic [3].
- A review of homoeopathic studies in the *British Medical Journal* in 2000 [4] suggested that homoeopath-prescribed preparations of individual's allergen may benefit symptoms.

References

1 Hay fever – practical management issues. *British Journal of General Practice* 2004; 54: 412 – 414
2 Common questions about hay fever. *MeReC Bulletin* Number 5, volume 14
3 Randomised controlled trial of butterbur and cetirizine for treating seasonal allergic rhinitis. *British Medical Journal* 2002; 324: 144 – 6
4 Randomised controlled trial of homoeopathy versus placebo in perennial allergic rhinitis with overview of four trial series. *British Medical Journal* 2000; 321: 471 – 476

Answer 8

Discuss how doctors can identify their learning needs.

Identification of learning needs forms the basis for personal learning plans, recommended both for personal learning and as a requirement for reappraisal. PLPs are individual. Lecture-based teaching suits some, and others learn best in small groups or by self-directed learning. PLPs allow the use of variety of learning styles to best suit personal style and needs.

Identification of learning needs

Consultation-based methods

- Patients' unmet needs (PUNS) and doctor's educational needs

(DENS).
- Clinical problems or queries prompt self-directed learning, eg looking up specific facts about a condition, its management, investigation and treatment.
- Patient follow-up may highlight failed treatment or poor understanding of the disease process. Patient questions may expose weaknesses, which may be difficult for the doctor. Bluffing, holding or honesty are all techniques used to gain time for information gathering.
- These enquiries may be prompted by the internet or media. Some doctors may resent this, while others embrace it as part of modern medicine.
- Joint surgeries allow us to learn how our colleagues manage their patients and allow sharing of consultation styles.
- Video consultations may highlight consultation problems and allow third party opinion.
- Patient questionnaires may reveal clinical and consultation learning needs.

Practice-based methods

- Conventional audit may show deficiencies in process of care and outcomes.
- Significant event audit may highlight deficiencies in systems and learning needs, eg missed diagnosis. These may then stimulate conventional audit to prevent further similar events. Sharing of positive and negative experiences, and reflection in a safe environment, make this a valuable tool.
- Staff feedback and practice meetings may allow all staff to point out areas of weakness in the others' knowledge base.
- Practice appraisals: comparison with other practices may allow identification of learning needs on both practice and personal levels.

Learning needs identified by patients

- Complaints may reveal learning needs, eg in delayed diagnosis as well as consultation needs and deficiencies in the process of care.
- Patient satisfaction surveys: provide confidential feedback on doctor's communication skills, attitudes and time-keeping.

Other sources

- Guidelines may differ from doctor's current management and stimulate research.

- Journals may highlight new ideas, which may stimulate learning. Some magazines eg *Pulse*, have update sections which refresh and appraise knowledge in certain areas.
- The internet may present new avenues of information for both doctors and patients, although these may need critical appraisal.
- The Prodigy system may highlight alternative management options in researching learning needs.
- Computer-based learning and assessment (eg the PEP CD) and internet distance learning appraisals (eg MCQs) may highlight areas for attention.
- Educational courses advertised in the medical press may be of relevance and assist learning.
- Visits to neighbouring or beacon practices may stimulate critical appraisal of our own work.

Ethical issues

- We have an ethical obligation to keep up to date, although we have autonomy in how we learn.
- Confidentiality issues need to be clarified, eg with significant event audits.

Answer 9

One of your practice nurses wishes to go on a course on screening for prostate cancer. What issues does this raise and how would you address her request?

Prostate cancer is the second commonest cause of male cancer death, with significant effects on quality of life; 60% of cases are metastatic at diagnosis. There is no consensus on whether screening or early aggressive treatment reduces mortality or morbidity. The practice nurse's request raises several important issues.

Why now?

- Why has she made the request?
- Significant event involving a missed diagnosis?
- A personal learning need in male health, eg stimulated by family or friend affected?
- Course advertised locally or run by the local PCO?
- Burnout: do courses allow a break from the practice?
- Are patients she sees in the practice asking her for screening?

Review current practice

- Counselling: who does this? The doctors or the practice nurse team?

- How is screening currently done? Digital examination or PSA or both?
- Over-75 health checks: Is there a need to discuss screening at these reviews?
- Review current guidelines. NICE guidance on referral for prostatism suggests offering men a PSA test with adequate counselling, but there is no national screening programme. No agreement on the best test but recent evidence suggests PSA should be combined with digital rectal examination.

Course issues

- Who is running it? Drug company sponsored or run by a local postgraduate centre?
- Any likely bias?

Financial issues

- Cost of the course.
- Costs of covering study leave or locum nurse.
- Increased investigations and referrals may result from positive screening results.

Practice issues

Employment issues

- Study leave: should be included in nurse contracts.
- Need budget for study leave, either allocated to individuals or shared with other staff.
- Equity issues: Is study leave shared equally? Colleagues will have to cover for absence and may compete for leave, eg for holidays. Is there a need for prioritising study leave based on the benefit to the practice?

Training issues

- Do the partners feel the course is necessary? Consider inviting a local urologist to discuss the issues with the practice staff as a whole.
- Digital rectal examination: Who will do it? Will course attendance by the nurse save GP appointments or create additional ones for rectal examinations?
- Is there a well-man clinic? Is this a good time to consider starting one if the nurse has identified a need? Does the practice have a high number of elderly patients? Consider offering screening at the

over-75 health check.
- Any PCT interest? Screening may increase secondary care referrals. Will the PCT fund the course?

Ethical issues

- Resources: Until screening is shown to be effective is it justified?
- Non-maleficence/beneficence: Harm may be prevented if screening detects disease which can be treated, but increased anxiety and side-effects from treatment and investigation in false positives may cause harm.
- Autonomy: Informed patients should be able to request or refuse screening.
- Consent: Informed consent, addressing the implications of a positive or negative result.
- Justice: Any screening programme should be offered to all the population to be targeted, not reserved for the worried, well-informed well.

Answer 10

Discuss the diagnosis and management of eating disorders. Give evidence to support your views.

Diagnosis

Only 1:10 people with eating disorders seek help [1], so be alert to possibility. NICE guidelines [2] suggest screening those at risk, eg low BMI or amenorrhoea, and triage into low/moderate risk and high risk to guide treatment. High-risk patients should be considered for inpatient care.

The SCOFF questionnaire is a simple screening tool [3], with high sensitivity and specificity:

- Do you make yourself **S**ick because you feel uncomfortably full?
- Do you worry you have lost **C**ontrol over how much you eat?
- Have you recently lost more than **O**ne stone in a 3-month period?
- Do you believe yourself to be **F**at when others say you are too thin?
- Would you say that **F**ood dominates your life?

  One point for every 'yes'; a score of 2 indicates a likely case of anorexia nervosa or bulimia.

  The *British Journal of General Practice* [4] suggested looking for personality clues, eg shyness, natural insecurity, alexithymia. DSM IV criteria should be used if in doubt. A *British Journal of General Practice* study [5] found wide variations in recognition and referral.

Management

Nutritional care

- For patients with anorexia, NICE guidelines suggest aiming for weight gain of 0.5 – 1.0 kg a week with multivitamin supplements and physical exercise.
- May need inpatient care.

Cognitive–behavioral therapy

- The NICE guidelines recommend psychological interventions such as CBT, analytic therapy, and interpersonal psychotherapy as first-line therapy. The guidance advocates a holistic approach in caring for people with eating disorders, eg including family therapy and dental care.
- One small study [6] found general practice-based treatment for bulimia with self-help booklets using CBT principles to be comparable with treatment in specialist clinic settings.
- A Cochrane systematic review [7] found some evidence for the efficacy of psychotherapy and CBT but stated that the studies had limitations, eg not blinded.
- *Clinical Evidence* concluded that CBT was likely to be beneficial both on its own and in combination with antidepressants, although again the studies were limited, eg blinding, different outcomes etc.

Drug therapy

- The *British Medical Journal* review of treatments for bulimia nervosa [8] suggested antidepressants can reduce bingeing and purging, and improve depression.
- Antidepressants and CBT are equally effective for bulimia nervosa, though drop-out rates are higher with antidepressants, due to their side-effects.
- An editorial in the *British Medical Journal* in 2004 [9] on treatment of anorexia nervosa emphasised need for nutritional support to ensure that vital organs are healthy, and suggested possible benefits from olanzapine and venlafaxine, although there may be problems with compliance.
- Care should be taken in anorexia not to use drugs that prolong the QT interval.
- Clinical evidence suggested that SSRIs can reduce bulimic symptoms in the short term. Doses often need to be significantly higher than usual eg 60 mg fluoxetine per day.
- There is some evidence from a meta-analysis [10] that combination

therapy of CBT plus SSRI is better than SSRI alone.

References

1   Sexual abuse and bulimia nervosa: three integrated case control comparisons. *American Journal of Psychiatry* 1994; 151: 402 – 407

2   *Eating disorders: Core interventions in the treatment and management of anorexia nervosa, bulimia nervosa and related eating disorders.* NICE Clinical Guideline 9. January 2004

3   The SCOFF questionnaire: assessment of a new screening tool for eating disorders. *British Medical Journal* 1999: 319; 1467 – 1468

4   Eating disordered patients: personality, alexithymia, and implications for primary health care. *British Journal of General Practice* 2000; 450: 21

5   Eating disorder service: GP referral to. Why the wide variation? *British Journal of General Practice* 2000; 50: 380 – 383

6   Specialist treatment versus self-help for bulimia nervosa: a randomised controlled trial in general practice. *British Journal of General Practice* 2003; 53: 371 – 377

7   *Cochrane Database of Systemic Reviews* 2000; (4): CD000562

8   Clinical review: extracts from best treatments. Bulimia nervosa. *British Medical Journal* 2003; 327: 380 – 383

9   Management of anorexia nervosa revisited [editorial]. *British Medical Journal* 2004; 328: 479 – 480

10 Combination of antidepressants and psychotherapy for bulimia nervosa: a systematic review. *Acta Psychiatrica Scandinavica* 2000; 101: 256 – 264

Answer 11

1   **What are the problems encountered in studying therapies in arthritis?**

- Problems may arise in identifying clinically relevant but objective outcome measures. Pain may be affected by many other variables as well as arthritis activity, such as depression, and this may act as a confounder.
- Symptoms often wax and wane, and apparent resolution may be a coincidence or due to a therapy under investigation.
- Clinical outcomes such as joint replacement may be decided on subjectively and this decision may be dependent on local resources, eg where there are long waiting lists for surgery it is less likely to be offered to patients.

See reference material 8.2a, an extract from the paper 'Long-term effects of glucosamine sulphate on osteoarthritis progression: a randomised, placebo-controlled clinical trial'. Reprinted with permission from Elsevier Science (*Lancet* 2001; 357: 251 – 256) and answer the following questions:

2   Comment on the methodology described in reference material 8.2a

- The trial was a randomised double blind placebo controlled trial, the gold standard clinical trial.
- Patients were included if they met formal diagnostic criteria for osteoarthritis, reducing the risk of confounding by other conditions (eg rheumatoid arthritis).
- X-rays were assessed automatically by a computer, avoiding bias in assessing outcomes.
- X-ray change is a surrogate outcome and may not reflect symptom frequency, however this was combined with symptom assessment by a validated system, the WOMAC score.
- The study sample size was calculated in advance to give sufficient power. The participants were selected from the outpatient clinic of a specialist centre, so they may not be representative of the general population, eg they may have severe osteoarthritis unresponsive to normal treatments. It is unclear how they were recruited, raising the possibility of inclusion bias, eg only certain groups being invited to join the study.
- Exclusion criteria included BMI > 30. Many patients with osteoarthritis will fall into this group and hence the results may not be applicable to patients seen in general practice.
- Randomisation was computerised, with sealed envelopes to blind the participants and examiners, avoiding inclusion/exclusion bias.
- The analysis was done on an intention-to-treat basis, making the results applicable to a clinical setting.
- The study was conducted over a 3-year period, sufficient to detect any effects.

3   Comment on the results in Tables 2 and 3 of reference material 8.2b

Table 2

- When patients taking the treatment for three years are compared with those taking placebo, there was no significant reduction in mean joint space or minimum joint space in the glucosamine group, with confidence intervals crossing 0.

- The placebo group had a statistically significant decrease, and the difference between placebo and glucosamine of 0.38 mm was significant with 95% confidence intervals of –0.17 to 0.32, p = 0.038.
- Similar results were obtained for minimum joint space narrowing. These statistically significant results persisted when intention-to-treat analysis was carried out, with p values < 0.05 for both mean and minimum joint space.

Table 3

- These results confirm a statistically significant difference of 34.1% (6.4 to 61.8%), p = 0.016 for patients completing the trial and 21.6% (3.5 to 39.6%) p = 0.020 for intention-to-treat.
- These confirm a benefit for WOMAC scores in patients taking glucosamine.

Answer 12

See reference material 8.3a, an extract from the paper 'The effect of GP telephone triage on numbers seeking same day appointments' (with copyright permission from *British Journal of General Practice* 2002; 52: 390–392). In terms of relevance to managing demand in UK general practice, discuss the methodology and results of this study.

Population

- The study was carried out in a market town in a practice with a list size of 7200. It is unclear whether it was the only practice in town or whether there was a minor illness unit in the town. Analysis of workload at these sites during the same period may show that patients offered telephone advice only simply went elsewhere for a face-to-face consultation.
- Jarman scores are given, but not ethnic mix. In areas with large ethnic communities in which English may not be spoken as a first language, the policy may be less effective.
- There is no mention of the age distribution of the population. This may affect the acceptability of the intervention. Younger patients may prefer to have telephone advice, avoiding a consultation, whereas the elderly may prefer the opposite.

Doctors

- No attempt was made to assess the satisfaction of the doctors with this form of triage. Many doctors find telephone triage stressful and prefer face-to-face consultations, particularly with children and patients they do not know.
- Do the partners have personal lists? Anecdotal evidence suggests patients are happier receiving, and doctors happier giving, telephone advice to people that they know.
- Was all the triage done by the duty doctor or by each doctor triaging their own patients?
- It is difficult to assess the impact of the drop in demand since only a percentage reduction is given rather than an actual figure for reduction in appointments or hours consulting saved. The time demands of telephone triage are approximately one hour a day. Does this reduce appointments by more than an hour a day? If not, the savings may be illusory.

Assessment

- Did the doctors know when they were going to have the patient satisfaction survey done? This may have introduced bias by the doctors modifying their behaviour.
- The method states that a patient satisfaction survey was sent to all patients who received a telephone call over a 1-month period. The results state that a 74% response rate with 111 responses was achieved, ie 150 questionnaires were sent out. The results go on to state that during the second half of the study, the average monthly call number was around 600. Did the workload increase four-fold between the two sampling periods? If so, the GP activity log should have been conducted on the same period as the satisfaction survey. Alternatively, did each person ring for a same-day appointment four times in the month, negating the benefits of the intervention in reducing demand? A third explanation is that the surveys were sent out to all callers over a 1-week period, not one month as reported in the paper.
- What was the effect on demand for routine appointments? Patients may have learnt that to be seen they need to ask for a routine rather than same-day appointment. Increased demand for routine appointments may cancel out any savings made in emergency appointments.
- No attempt was made to compare doctor triage with nurse triage. GPs are an expensive commodity to use for telephone triage. It may be that nurses could provide a similar service at lower cost.

Financial costs

- Any other financial costs? Tying up an outside line for triage for one hour a day may block incoming calls, requiring further investment in hardware.
- Did prescribing change before and after the intervention? Prescriptions were offered in   . % of consultations. A large proportion of these presumably were for antibiotics, telephone prescribing of which is frowned upon by the Standing Advisory Committee. Increased prescribing costs may remove any benefit in reduced appointments.

Abbreviations

A&E	Accident and Emergency
ACE	acetylcholine esterase
AF	atrial fibrillation
ARR	absolute risk reduction
BHF	British Heart Foundation
BMA	British Medical Association
BMI	body mass index
BNF	British National Formulary
BP	blood pressure
BTS	British Thoracic Society
CBT	cognitive behavioural therapy
CDH	congenital dislocation of the hip
CHImp	Commission for Health Improvement
CNS	central nervous system
COCP	combined oral contraceptive pill
COPD	chronic obstructive pulmonary disease
COX 2	cyclo-oxygenase 2
CPN	community psychiatric nurse
CRP	C-reactive protein
CT	computed tomography
CVS	cardiovascular system
DCCT	Diabetes Control and Complications Trial
DENS	doctor's educational needs
DEXA	dual energy x-ray absorptiometry
DGH	district general hospital
DM	diabetes mellitus
DNA	deoxyribonucleic acid
DNA	did not attend
DOH	Department of Health
DSM	IV APA Diagnostic and Statistical Manual, 4th edition
DVLA	Driver and Vehicle Licensing Authority
DVT	deep venous thrombosis
ECG	electrocardiogram
ENT	ear, nose and throat
ESR	erythrocyte sedimentation rate
FBC	full blood count
FEV_1	forced expiratory volume in one second

FSH	follicle stimulating hormone
GI	gastrointestinal
GMC	General Medical Council
GMS	General Medical Services
GORD	gastro-oesophageal reflux disease
GPwSI	General Practitioner with special interest
GUM	genito-urinary medicine
H2RA	H2 receptor antagonist
HOPE	Heart Outcomes Prevention Evaluation
HDL	high density lipoproteins
HIV	human immunodeficiency virus
HRT	hormone replacement therapy
HVS	high vaginal swab
IBS	irritable bowel syndrome
ICU	intensive care unit
IHD	ischaemic heart disease
INR	International Normalized Ratio
IOS	items of service
IPSO	Ibuprofen, Paracetamol Study in Osteoarthritis
LDL	low-density lipoproteins
LFT	liver function test
LH	luteinising hormone
LMC	local medical committee
LMP	last menstrual period
LV	left ventricle
MDU	Medical Defence Union
MI	myocardial infarction
MMR	measles, mumps and rubella vaccination
MMTS	mini mental test score
MND	motor neurone disease
MRSA	methicillin-resistant *Staphylococcus aureus*
MS	multiple sclerosis
nGMS	new General Medical Services
NICE	National Institute for Clinical Excellence
NNT	number needed to treat
NSAID	non-steroidal anti-inflammatory drug
NSF	National Service Framework
OA	osteoarthritis
OAE	otoacoustic emission
OT	occupational therapy
PACT	Prescribing Analysis and Cost
PCG	primary care group
PCO	primary care organisation
PCT	primary care trust

PHCT	primary healthcare trust
PLP	personal learning plan
PMS	Personal Medical Services
PPI	proton-pump inhibitor
PSA	prostate specific antigen
PTSD	post-traumatic stress disorder
PUNS	patients' unmet needs
PVS	persistent vegetative state
RCN	Royal College of Nurses
RCT	randomised controlled trial
RNIB	Royal National Institute for the Blind
RR	relative risk
SERM	selective oestrogen receptor modulator
SLE	systemic lupus erythematosus
SSRI	selective serotonin re-uptake inhibitor
STD	sexually transmitted disease
TFT	thyroid function test
TIA	transient ischaemic attack
TURP	transurethral
UKPDS	United Kingdom Prospective Diabetes Study
WHO	World Health Organization
WOMAC	Western Ontario and McMaster Universities

Index

Riluzole
Naltrexon ⟩ dedduto
Acamprosat ⟩
Trimerosal — nauceo
Risperidone — antipsychotic
Seloken — coprolu Dementia
Doneptzil
riventyni
Xilulofotin